THE ULTIMATE LOW-FODMAP DIET

GUIDE & COOKBOOK

LEARN TO MANAGE AND SOOTHE IBS AND OTHER DIGESTIVE DISORDERS WITH QUICK, TASTY, NUTRITIOUS MEALS. INCLUDES A 28-DAY MEAL PLAN, ALSO VEGGIE

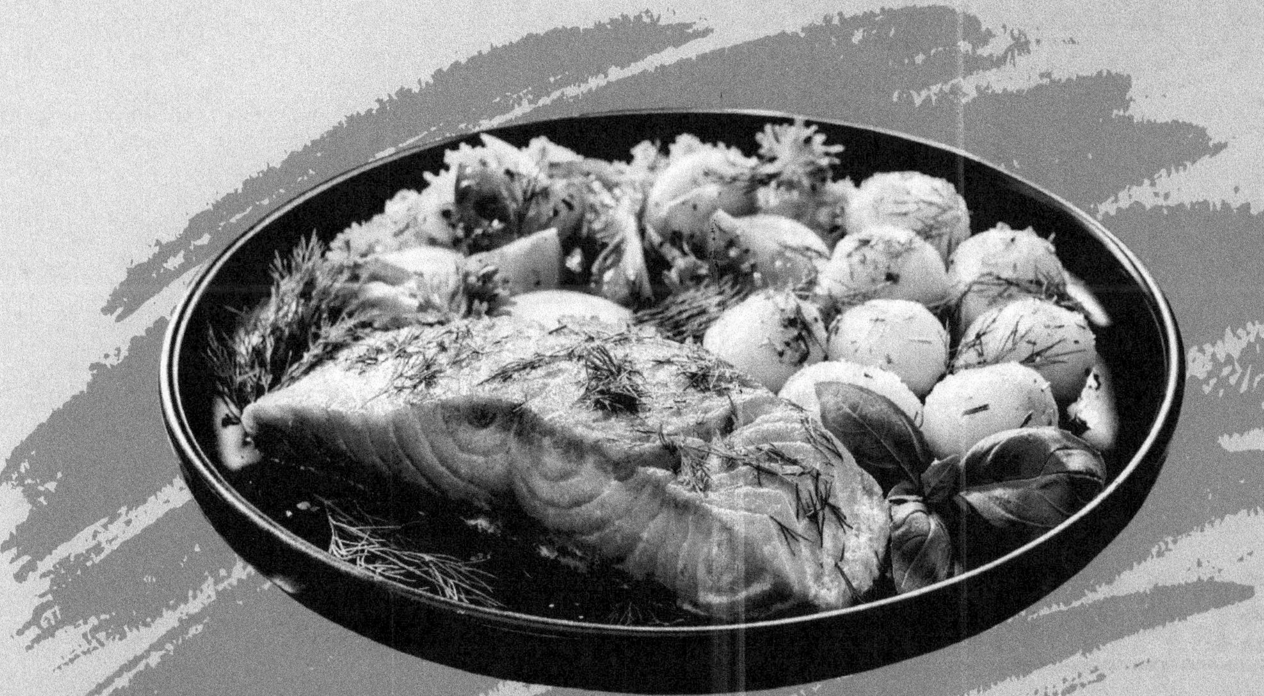

Kate Bloom

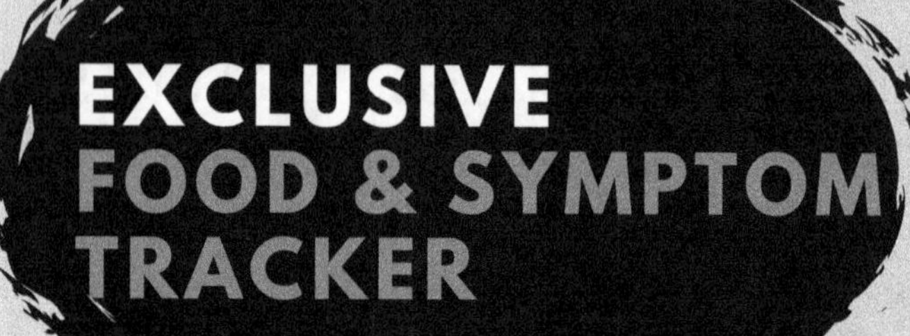

THANK YOU FOR PURCHASING MY BOOK!

IF YOU ENJOYED IT, I WOULD APPRECIATE YOUR HONEST FEEDBACK ON AMAZON

If you have any concerns, please email me at:

info@topqualitybooks.com

I want to create high-quality products that give everyone satisfaction

AUTHOR PAGE

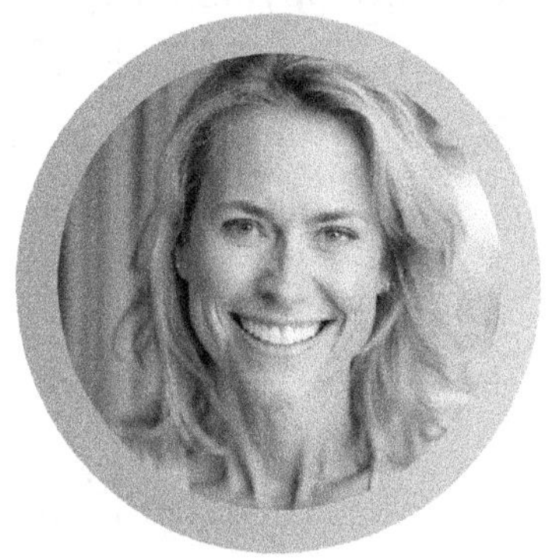

Kate Bloom, a nutrition and wellness specialist, has devoted her career to aiding individuals to lead healthier lives free from the symptoms of various gastrointestinal disorders. A staunch advocate for the healing properties of food, Kate has combined her personal journey and professional expertise to publish guides, cookbooks, and tailored food plans. Her work offers hope to millions worldwide who face daily challenges with these health issues.

Coming from a family of medical professionals, Kate has always been fascinated by the complexities of human health. However, her true calling emerged from her health struggles as a teenager. During a time typically marked by carefree attitudes and fun, Kate contended with persistent heartburn, acid reflux, and emerging digestive problems that severely impacted her social life.

Since those early challenges, Kate has been relentlessly questing to understand the connection between nutrition and health. Her mission is straightforward: empowering others to control their health and well-being. She achieves this by sharing her knowledge, life experiences, and culinary skills. Her writing is insightful, intentionally straightforward, and direct, aiming to simplify complex nutritional concepts for her readers and provide practical, actionable advice.

Today, Kate enjoys a life free from the symptoms that once plagued her, a testament to the efficacy of the strategies and recipes she advocates in her books. In her leisure time, she continues to experiment with new recipes, determined to prove that dietary restrictions don't have to mean bland and uninteresting meals.

Kate Bloom

INTRODUCTION

The human digestive system, a series of interconnected organs from mouth to anus, serves as the body's nutritional highway—a pivotal roadway for overall health and well-being. Healthy digestion and maintaining heart and bone health are cornerstones of general bodily health, with proper gut function immensely impacting daily living.

Digestion is a complex process of transformation whereby food is converted into nutrients to nourish the body. This intricate process fuels the body's billions of cells, which form everything from your skin and bones to muscles and organs. A healthy digestive process means you are unlikely to suffer from unpleasant symptoms such as heartburn, gas, constipation, diarrhea, nausea, or stomach discomfort, which can impede everyday activities.

One might be surprised to learn that digestion begins as soon as food enters the mouth and does not conclude until it ends in the small intestine. The digestive system, often overlooked unless it is causing discomfort, plays a critical role in the body's functioning. Its primary task is to break down food and assist in nutrient absorption, which has far-reaching effects on overall health, influencing everything from complexion to hair quality and sleep patterns.

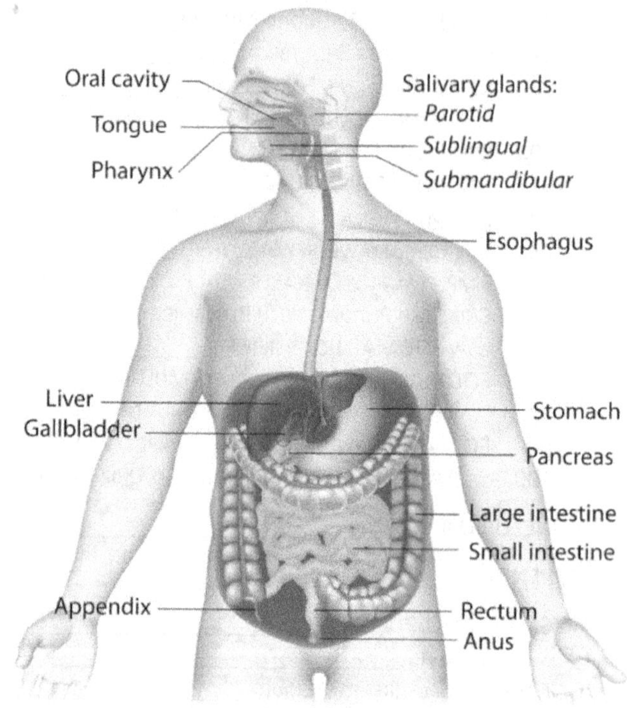

When the digestive system is not functioning optimally, symptoms can range from weight fluctuation and nausea to bloating and constipation, significantly impacting one's quality of life. On a broader level, digestive health can affect the ability to work, exercise, and socialize.

The small intestine takes the baton from the stomach in this relay of digestion, performing the majority of digestive work. The liver, a versatile organ, processes nutrients absorbed from the intestine, storing some for future use and distributing others to where they are immediately needed. The residual waste then proceeds to the large intestine and is eventually expelled from the body.

Maintaining a healthy digestive system is of utmost importance, and we cannot overstate the significance of diet in achieving this. The low-FODMAP diet, for instance, promotes positive impacts on digestion, health, and overall well-being, demonstrating that dieting does not always need to be a stressful endeavor. By incorporating creative thinking and simple hacks, pursuing a healthier diet can be enjoyable rather than a chore.

In the grand scheme, the digestive system serves as the body's "engine," powering the human body's complex machinery. When functioning optimally, it is a sophisticated system that allows the body to extract nutrients and energy from our food. The digestive process is not merely a means to an end; it plays a significant role in ensuring the body functions as it should. Hence, the saying "you are what you eat" emphasizes the importance of good nutrition and reminds us never to disregard our "gut feelings."

It's essential to recognize that many people worldwide, about 20% of the population, deal with gastrointestinal issues. These can result in symptoms like stomach bloating, fullness, discomfort, flatulence, or changes in bowel movements, indicating conditions such as Irritable Bowel Syndrome (IBS) and Functional Gastrointestinal Disorders (FGID). While the causes of these conditions are unknown, strategies like the low-FODMAP diet have effectively alleviated these symptoms.

The low-FODMAP diet, created by researchers at Monash University in Australia, offers hope to those experiencing discomfort. It aims to identify and avoid foods that cause pain. FODMAPs—Fermentable Oligosaccharides, Disaccharides, Monosaccharides, and Polyols—are a group of carbohydrates that can trigger IBS symptoms due to poor absorption in the small intestine and subsequent fermentation in the gut, leading to discomfort, bloating, and altered bowel movements.

The diet consists of three phases: elimination, reintroduction, and personalization. It begins with removing high-FODMAP foods such as onions, garlic, wheat, and certain fruits from the diet, followed by their gradual reintroduction to identify personal triggers. The final phase involves personalizing the diet based on individual responses, allowing individuals to regain control over their health and symptoms. This diet reduces symptoms and enhances dietary awareness, which improves overall quality of life.

Nevertheless, it's essential to consult a healthcare professional before significantly changing your diet or lifestyle. Your doctor can help rule out other significant intestinal conditions with similar symptoms, guide the low-FODMAP diet and its potential benefits for your specific condition, and ensure you receive the necessary support and guidance on your journey to better digestive health.

The low-FODMAP diet helps many people with digestive issues feel better without relying on medications or experiencing potential side effects. Through this targeted approach, individuals can discover new foods that they previously believed caused discomfort but can now be a safe and enjoyable part of their diet.

Each person's experience with gastrointestinal diseases and their response to the low-FODMAP diet is unique. As our understanding of the low-FODMAP diet evolves, it promises to remain a valuable tool in managing IBS and others, offering hope and relief to affected individuals.

Here are some of the common digestive disorders.

The IBS

Irritable Bowel Syndrome (IBS) is a prevalent chronic gastrointestinal disorder that significantly impacts the quality of life for numerous individuals. Common symptoms include abdominal pain, variations in stool consistency, incomplete bowel movements, mucus in the stool, and worsening symptoms following meals. IBS presents with periods of remission (when symptoms are mild or absent) and flare-ups (when symptoms are severe or worsen) and is classified into IBS-C (constipation-predominant), IBS-D (diarrhea-predominant), and IBS-A (alternating between constipation and diarrhea). Although the exact etiology of IBS is not fully understood, it is believed to involve multiple factors, including stress. Heightened intestinal sensitivity due to increased permeability of the intestinal lining is considered to contribute to IBS symptoms.

While the precise cause of IBS remains elusive, potential triggers encompass dietary factors, stress, and hormonal changes. It's important to acknowledge the validity of personal experiences and the tangible nature of this condition, particularly the role of stress. Certain food groups, such as wheat, dairy products, citrus fruits, and specific carbohydrates known as FODMAPs, may exacerbate IBS symptoms. While stress does not directly cause IBS, it can notably trigger or worsen symptoms. Hormonal changes, particularly prevalent in women, might also play a role in the development of IBS.

Diagnosis of IBS relies on symptom manifestation and excludes other gastrointestinal disorders, as there is no specific diagnostic test. Management involves symptom control through dietary modifications, medications such as antispasmodics, laxatives, antidepressants, probiotics, and stress management techniques. While specific nutritional elements may provoke or exacerbate symptoms, a balanced, nutrient-rich diet is fundamental for overall health and promoting a healthy gut environment. However, individual responses to dietary changes can vary, highlighting the importance of comprehending unique reactions to different foods. Managing IBS can pose challenges, but effective strategies such as a low-FODMAP diet can significantly enhance the quality of life. There is hope for improved quality of life through appropriate management strategies.

Functional Gastrointestinal Disorders (FGIDs)

Functional Gastrointestinal Disorders (FGIDs) denote conditions characterized by altered digestive sensitivity and motor activities without identifiable organic pathology. These functional alterations can manifest in any segment of the gastrointestinal tract. Prevalent in Western countries, FGIDs afflict 15-20% of the population and give rise to unpredictable symptoms that substantially impact patients' quality of life. Consequently, affected individuals frequently seek medical attention, undergo diagnostic procedures, resort to medication, and may even undergo unnecessary surgeries. While these disorders do not precipitate physical degeneration or reduce life expectancy, they diminish overall well-being. Primarily prevalent in women, FGIDs can affect individuals across all age groups, including children.

Clinical presentations commonly encompass heartburn, retrosternal chest pain, dysphagia, dyspepsia, cyclic vomiting syndrome, abdominal pain, and irritable bowel syndrome. Diagnostic protocols hinge on symptomatic assessment once organic pathologies have been excluded. Although standardized therapeutic modalities are lacking, specialists advocate tailored interventions comprising dietary modifications, pharmacotherapeutic agents targeting diverse aspects of gastrointestinal and nervous system function, and practical lifestyle adjustments.

Crohn's Disease

Crohn's disease is a serious, chronic inflammatory condition that can affect any part of the digestive system. If left untreated, it can lead to intestinal ulcers and serious complications such as stenosis or fistulas. Common symptoms include abdominal pain, persistent diarrhea, weight loss, and fever. About 90% of patients experience the disease in the small intestine and colon. While the exact cause is not fully understood, a combination of factors, including genetic predisposition, environmental influences such as diet and exposure to specific pathogens, smoking, and changes in the intestinal flora and immune response, are believed to contribute to its development.

The symptoms of Crohn's disease can present wide variability depending on its location within the body. However, typical indicators consist of chronic diarrhea, abdominal pain, cramps, blood in stool, weight loss, low-grade fever, and occasionally joint pain. The disease may not always manifest with symptoms so that it may be incidentally discovered. This unpredictability highlights the necessity of comprehensive diagnostic methods, encompassing colonoscopy with ileum visualization and biopsy, ultrasonography of the intestinal loops, abdominal MRI, and, occasionally, surgical exploration under anesthesia.

The management of Crohn's disease focuses on reducing intestinal inflammation with personalized therapy to address the patient's symptoms. While it's not possible to prevent the disease, effective management relies on early detection and regular monitoring. This proactive approach can help prevent complications and slow the disease's progression. It involves regular blood and stool tests, non-invasive abdominal exams, and frequent colonoscopies to detect any signs of intestinal neoplasia in advanced cases of colonic disease.

<u>**Celiac Disease**</u>

Celiac disease is an inherited inflammatory condition that primarily affects the mucosa of the small intestine. It triggers an immune response to gluten, wheat, barley, and rye protein. This disease can develop at any age and is often associated with other autoimmune conditions such as type 1 diabetes, rheumatoid arthritis, and thyroid disease.

When genetically predisposed individuals consume gluten, their immune cells attack the mucosa of the small intestine, causing damage to the villi responsible for nutrient absorption. This leads to malabsorption and malnutrition. Celiac disease affects around 1% of the population, with a higher prevalence among women, and many cases go undiagnosed.

Symptoms can vary widely. The "classical form" often presents at an early age with malabsorption symptoms like foul-smelling diarrhea, abdominal cramping, and slow growth. Conversely, the more common "atypical form" can occur in adults with nonspecific symptoms such as anemia, osteoporosis, muscle fatigue, fertility issues, and coagulation problems.

Doctors initially conduct a blood test to diagnose celiac disease and check for specific antibodies produced in response to gluten. If the test is positive, a duodenal biopsy is performed to confirm villi damage. Genetic testing may also be considered in uncertain cases. Due to the hereditary nature of the disease, the patient's first-degree relatives should undergo screening. Despite its widespread prevalence, people can effectively manage celiac disease with a gluten-free diet.

<u>**Small Intestinal Bacterial Overgrowth (SIBO)**</u>

Small Intestinal Bacterial Overgrowth (SIBO) is a complex condition marked by excessive bacteria growth or the presence of abnormal bacteria in the small intestine. This part of the intestine is responsible for the absorption of most nutrients and typically has significantly fewer bacteria than the large intestine. SIBO disrupts the balance in the small intestine, with bacteria either overpopulating or migrating from the colon, resulting in various unpleasant symptoms.

Diagnosing SIBO can be a puzzle as the symptoms often mimic those of several other conditions. These include diarrhea, abdominal bloating, chronic abdominal pain, and, in severe cases, malabsorption of vitamin B12 leading to anemia. It is of utmost importance to distinguish SIBO from other conditions, such as gastritis, irritable bowel syndrome, allergies, and intolerances, to ensure accurate diagnosis and effective treatment.

The diagnosis of SIBO typically involves a non-invasive Lactulose Breath Test, a valuable tool in our diagnostic arsenal. During this test, the patient breathes into a bag before and after consuming synthetic sugar lactulose. Bacterial fermentation of lactulose in the gut leads to an increase in the hydrogen content of exhaled air. Typically, peaks in breath hydrogen occur between 30 and 90 minutes; deviations from this range may indicate disorders affecting regular intestinal transit. By following specific guidelines, this test can provide invaluable insights into the patient's gut health and potential imbalances, thereby aiding in the diagnosis and treatment of SIBO.

<u>**Ulcerative Colitis**</u>

Ulcerative colitis is a chronic inflammatory bowel disease characterized by long-lasting inflammation of the intestinal walls, often leading to symptoms such as bloody diarrhea, discomfort, fatigue, and weight loss. The condition typically starts in the rectum and can spread to the first part of the colon. Besides affecting the gastrointestinal tract, ulcerative colitis can also impact other areas, such as the joints, skin, and eyes. It has periods of remission and exacerbation.

The specific cause of ulcerative colitis is still unknown. People believe an inappropriate immune response to environmental factors within the intestines, particularly in individuals with a genetic predisposition, causes it. Risk factors for the condition may include age, race, and family history. Individuals can develop ulcerative colitis at any age, but doctors most commonly diagnose it before the age of 30. It is more common in white individuals and those of Ashkenazi Jewish descent.

Diagnosing ulcerative colitis usually requires a thorough assessment, including clinical, endoscopic, histological, and radiological examinations, along with a detailed review of the patient's medical history. Adopting a healthy lifestyle and dietary habits can help manage symptoms and extend periods of remission. Patients often receive advice to consider making nutritional changes such as limiting dairy and high-fat foods, reducing fiber intake, avoiding spicy foods, consuming smaller meals, staying hydrated, and considering multivitamins. Moreover, quitting smoking is highly recommended, as it is a confirmed lifestyle-related risk factor.

Despite the chronic nature of ulcerative colitis, individuals can lead an everyday life with appropriate management and treatment. However, the persistent inflammation associated with the condition can increase the risk of colorectal cancer, emphasizing the importance of regular medical check-ups and preventive measures.

.

Low-FODMAP Diet

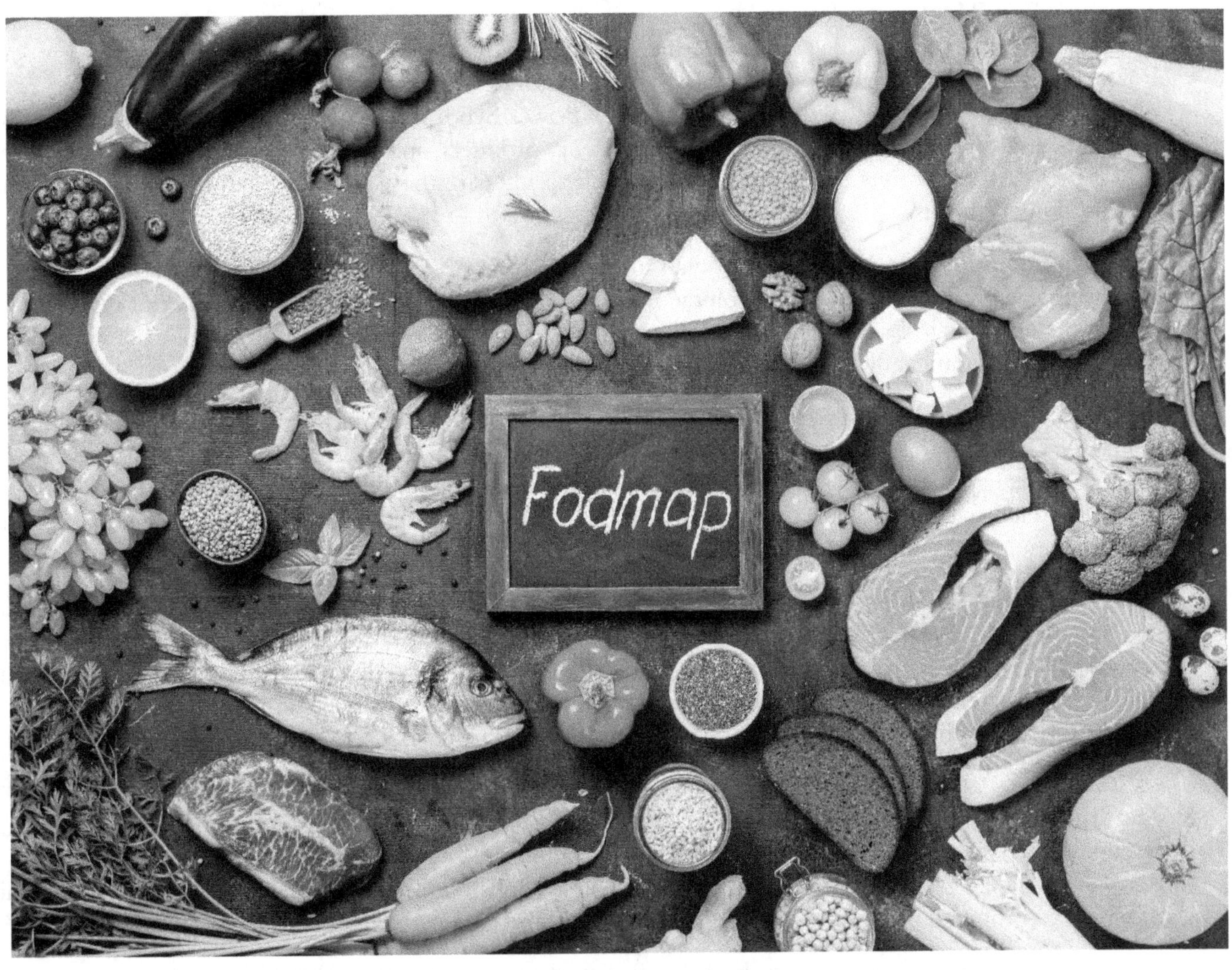

The Low-FODMAP diet, designed to alleviate digestive discomfort, is backed by substantial scientific research and based on understanding Fermentable Oligosaccharides, Disaccharides, Monosaccharides, and Polyols (FODMAPs). These specific types of carbohydrates, found in various foods, are known to cause digestive issues, especially in those with Irritable Bowel Syndrome (IBS). High-FODMAP foods include apples, wheat, onions, garlic, legumes, lactose-rich dairy products, and sweeteners like sorbitol and xylitol. The Low-FODMAP diet offers a personalized approach to mitigate these discomforts by reducing the intake of high-FODMAP foods.

When you consume FODMAPs, your small intestine poorly absorbs them, and gut bacteria ferment them, increasing gas production and water volume in the gut. This rapid fermentation process can result in various symptoms, including bloating, gas, stomach pain, constipation, and diarrhea. For individuals with IBS, these symptoms can significantly affect their quality of life.

Researchers at Monash University in Australia pioneered the low-FODMAP diet, a significant development in managing IBS symptoms. This diet, operating in three phases: elimination, reintroduction, and maintenance, aims to reduce symptoms by gradually lowering the intake of high-FODMAP foods and reintroducing them in a controlled manner to identify trigger foods. This diet's research and practical application have shown effective results in managing IBS symptoms and improving patients' quality of life.

Numerous clinical trials and studies supporting the effectiveness of this diet have demonstrated the benefits of a low-FODMAP diet for managing IBS symptoms. According to a landmark study at Monash University, around 70% of IBS patients experienced significant symptom relief when following a low-FODMAP diet. A systematic review and meta-analysis of multiple studies published in the "Journal of Gastroenterology" has reinforced these findings, revealing a considerable reduction in IBS symptoms, including abdominal pain, bloating, and bowel habit abnormalities.

The effectiveness of the Low-FODMAP diet is not only supported by scientific research but also recognized by numerous reputable gastroenterological organizations worldwide. These include the British Dietetic Association, the American College of Gastroenterology, and the Gastroenterological Society of Australia, all of which recommend the Low-FODMAP diet as a first-line therapy for managing IBS symptoms.

It's important to note that the Low-FODMAP diet, despite its benefits, should be implemented under the supervision of a healthcare professional or registered dietitian. This personalized guidance is crucial to ensure the diet is followed correctly, maximizes symptom relief, and maintains nutritional balance.

Looking at the list of high-FODMAP foods, it becomes clear that healthy and unhealthy foods can fall into this category. The common denominator between these foods is the presence of carbohydrates, including simple and complex carbs and fiber. When these carbohydrates reach the stomach, they ferment, resulting in bloating and discomfort if the stomach's bacteria are disrupted or the meal remains in the gut for too long.

It is worth noting that some individuals with a functional digestive disorder may be unable to digest certain carbohydrates properly. This malabsorption results in an overabundance of food for the bacteria in the large intestine, leading to rapid fermentation that produces acids, alcohol, and carbon dioxide. This process can alter the gut's pH and cause various symptoms, ranging from gas and belching to inflammation and acid reflux.

Moreover, these FODMAPs are osmotic, which can attract and retain water. While this property can be advantageous in some contexts (like keeping baked goods moist), it can cause bloating and discomfort when sensitive individuals consume high-FODMAP foods.

The Low-FODMAP diet, introduced in 2001, has been a beacon of hope for many suffering from IBS. While it took time for research to back up its effectiveness, an increasing number of individuals have found significant relief from IBS symptoms by avoiding high-FODMAP foods. Through scientific backing and practical application, the low-FODMAP diet has proven to be a vital tool in managing IBS and providing a renewed sense of comfort and relief for millions of individuals worldwide.

The low-FODMAP diet operates on the principle of reducing and controlling the intake of dietary FODMAPs. FODMAPs, as explained in the previous chapter, are an acronym for Fermentable Oligosaccharides, Disaccharides, Monosaccharides, and Polyols. They are poorly absorbed carbohydrates in the gut. When they reach the colon, they ferment and increase the stomach's water volume, thereby causing typical IBS symptoms such as bloating, gas, and altered bowel movements.

The implementation of a Low-FODMAP diet entails traversing through three critical phases:

- **Elimination;**
- **Reintroduction;**
- **Maintenance.**

Each phase aims to help identify the foods that trigger IBS symptoms, develop a personalized and sustainable diet plan, and ensure long-term symptom management.

The elimination phase, marking the start of the low-FODMAP diet, involves removing all high-FODMAP foods from the diet for a period, typically between 2 and 6 weeks. The intention here is to allow the gut to 'reset,' reducing inflammation and the symptoms associated with IBS. Due to the highly restrictive nature of the diet during this period, this phase should ideally be completed under the supervision of a dietitian or healthcare professional.

The subsequent reintroduction phase, initiated after the elimination phase, involves gradually reintroducing high-FODMAP foods back into the diet, one at a time. This phase is crucial as it allows the identification of specific foods or groups of foods that trigger your symptoms. This is of utmost importance as everyone's response to different FODMAPs can vary greatly. Some might react to fructans, others to lactose or polyols, while others might find they are tolerant to specific amounts of some FODMAPs.

Following the reintroduction phase, the maintenance or personalization phase begins. Here, the diet is tailored to avoid only the specific FODMAPs that are known to trigger your symptoms, thus allowing you to enjoy a varied diet without the discomfort typically associated with IBS.

Overall, the low-FODMAP diet reduces the dietary load of these fermentable carbohydrates, thus decreasing their fermentation and water-drawing effects in the gut. This approach allows for better control and management of IBS symptoms, improving quality of life.

The diet aims not to eliminate FODMAPs but to identify which ones trigger your symptoms. It is also essential to ensure that a wide range of nutrients is included in your diet to maintain overall health.

Implementing the Low-FODMAP diet can be challenging, and professional guidance is often crucial for its success. A dietitian or healthcare professional can provide invaluable advice, from ensuring nutritional adequacy to providing support and motivation. They can help you navigate the distinct phases, maintain a balanced diet, and answer any questions.

The Low-FODMAP diet is not a one-size-fits-all solution. It is about understanding your body's responses and adapting the diet to suit your unique needs and lifestyle. By personalizing your diet, planning your meals, getting creative with recipes, and prioritizing variety, you can make the Low-FODMAP diet work for you. Most importantly, listen to your body. If a particular food causes discomfort, it is okay to avoid it. Conversely, suppose you can tolerate a traditionally high food in FODMAPs. In that case, there is no need to eliminate it from your diet.

Embarking on the Low-FODMAP diet is a journey towards better managing your IBS symptoms. Understanding and successfully navigating each diet phase is vital to this journey. With the correct information, guidance, and a commitment to listening to your body, the low-FODMAP diet can help you improve your digestive health and overall quality of life.

STRATEGIES FOR REINTRODUCING HIGH-FODMAP FOODS

The initial elimination phase of the Low-FODMAP diet reduces IBS symptoms, but you should not follow it indefinitely. The subsequent reintroduction phase allows for the careful reincorporation of some high-FODMAP foods back into your diet. This process enables the identification of specific FODMAPs that trigger your symptoms, leading to a more personalized and varied diet plan that maximizes nutritional adequacy.

During the reintroduction phase, one category of FODMAPs is brought back at a time, symptoms are monitored, and results are recorded. This task may seem daunting, but with a structured plan and the invaluable guidance of a dietitian, it becomes an efficient process of gathering valuable data about your personal FODMAP tolerance levels. The reintroduction phase can last several weeks or months, depending on your response to different FODMAPs.

Before beginning the reintroduction process, establish a baseline of minimal symptoms. Gradually reintroducing high-FODMAP foods provides a clear basis for comparison. Preparing for reintroduction also involves maintaining a detailed food and symptom diary, understanding the reintroduction process and what it entails, mentally preparing for the potential return of IBS symptoms, and considering seeking professional guidance to navigate the operation efficiently.

Planning your reintroduction requires choosing one FODMAP group to reintroduce at a time, selecting a high-FODMAP food that contains that FODMAP exclusively, gradually increasing the serving size of that food over time, and monitoring your body's reaction to the reintroduced food. This meticulous approach, guided by a dietitian, can provide personalized advice on which foods to reintroduce and in what order based on your unique nutritional needs and preferences.

Monitoring symptoms during reintroduction is crucial to accurately identifying triggers. Keep a detailed record of the food and serving size consumed, the time of consumption, and any resulting symptoms. Take note of emerging patterns and understand that symptoms may not always occur immediately after eating a high-FODMAP food. Symptoms can be delayed up to 48 hours, and other factors like stress, hormonal changes, or physical activity can also influence IBS symptoms. This heightened self-awareness is key to your success in managing your IBS symptoms.

Once you have reintroduced a high-FODMAP food and noted any symptoms, interpreting your results is a crucial step that informs your long-term diet plan. It's important to assess the severity, duration, and onset of symptoms, consider the quantity of the food consumed, and not rush to label a food as a trigger prematurely. Remember, this is a process that requires patience and thoroughness. Seeking guidance from a dietitian can help interpret results and design a long-term diet plan that is nutritionally balanced and symptom-managing.

Embarking on the reintroduction phase of high-FODMAP foods is a significant step towards taking control of your IBS symptoms in the long term. It's a journey that transitions you from a strictly low-FODMAP diet to a more flexible and personalized approach, enhancing dietary variety and nutritional adequacy. Remember, everyone's tolerance to different FODMAPs varies, and this process is about learning about your unique triggers rather than comparing your experiences to others. This knowledge will empower you to create a customized diet that effectively manages your symptoms while allowing you to enjoy a wide range of foods.

The ultimate goal of the Low-FODMAP diet is to empower you to develop a personalized eating plan after the reintroduction phase that maximizes food variety and minimizes IBS symptoms. This means your long-term diet should be based on your tolerance levels for FODMAPs identified during the reintroduction phase.

Your diet should primarily consist of low-FODMAP foods, and high-FODMAP foods should be reintroduced successfully without causing significant symptoms. At the same time, foods that trigger symptoms should be limited or avoided. It's essential to continue monitoring for any signs as your tolerance to certain FODMAPs may change. Experimenting with portion sizes may also help you expand your diet to include a broader range of foods without discomfort.

While managing IBS symptoms is a priority, it's equally important to maintain your overall health. A vital aspect of a long-term low-FODMAP diet is to ensure that it is not only low in FODMAPs but also nutritionally balanced. This means it should include various food groups to meet all your nutritional needs. By emphasizing this balance, you can feel confident that you're not just managing your IBS, but also taking care of your overall health.

Consider seeking continued professional support from a dietitian or healthcare provider. They can help manage any new or recurring symptoms and provide personalized advice for your long-term dietary strategy. Remember, the low-FODMAP diet is not just a diet; it's a journey of self-discovery. It's a tool that can help you understand your body better, identify your trigger foods, and find a dietary balance that suits your unique needs. Successfully navigating the reintroduction phase with these strategies, under the guidance of a professional, will assist you in developing a personalized long-term dietary plan that manages your IBS symptoms while meeting your nutritional needs.

LOW-FODMAP DIET FOR FOOD INTOLERANCES/ALLERGIES AND VEGETARIAN LIFESTYLES

The low-FODMAP diet can accommodate various dietary needs, including food allergies, celiac disease, lactose intolerance, nut allergies, and vegetarian or vegan lifestyles. However, to effectively implement this diet, it's crucial to understand the nature of FODMAPs, which are present in various food groups.

Specific food intolerances, such as lactose and fructose intolerance, are directly related to FODMAPs. The low-FODMAP diet can naturally benefit individuals with these intolerances by reducing the intake of high-lactose dairy products and fructose-rich fruits and sweeteners. However, it's important to note that those with a milk protein allergy might still have adverse reactions to lactose-free dairy substitutes, so they may need to opt for plant-based alternatives.

For individuals with celiac disease, an autoimmune disorder triggered by gluten, the Low-FODMAP diet must exclude all gluten-containing grains, regardless of their FODMAP content. Gluten-free grains like rice, quinoa, and oats become substitutes for wheat, barley, and rye. Moreover, it's essential to use separate cooking utensils, clean surfaces thoroughly, and carefully read food labels for hidden sources of gluten to avoid cross-contamination with gluten-containing foods.

In the case of food allergies, such as nut allergies, it's important to avoid the allergen, even if the offending food is low in FODMAPs. Incorporating alternatives like seeds and other protein sources into the diet does not worsen IBS symptoms.

Adapting the low-FODMAP diet to vegetarian and vegan lifestyles may seem challenging because some staple plant-based foods are high in FODMAPs. However, with careful planning, it is entirely feasible. For instance, protein sources such as firm tofu, tempeh, and canned lentils or chickpeas can be excellent choices in small quantities. It's important to note that while these are low-FODMAP alternatives, consuming them in large amounts may still trigger IBS symptoms, so portion control is critical.

Adapting common vegetarian foods for a low-FODMAP diet can be a fun and creative challenge. You can swap high-FODMAP grains with low-FODMAP alternatives, adjust seasonings, substitute legumes, revise vegetables and fruits, and monitor your portions. Over time, with some creativity and experimentation, you can manage your IBS symptoms and enjoy flavorful, satisfying meals. This possibility should fill you with hope and positivity as you navigate your dietary restrictions.

Successfully managing IBS symptoms depends on understanding your unique nutritional requirements, planning meals carefully, modifying recipes, and being creative in your cooking. Regardless of specific dietary needs or lifestyle choices, the goal is to manage your symptoms while enjoying your food effectively.

In conclusion, keeping a food diary can help identify personal triggers and tailor the low-FODMAP diet to your needs. To do this effectively, you must record what you eat and the portion sizes, preparation methods, and any symptoms you experience. The journal can help you track your food intake, symptoms, and any patterns between them. This insight can be particularly beneficial when managing multiple dietary considerations.

COMBINING A LOW-FODMAP AND HIGH-PROTEIN DIET

To maintain an active lifestyle often means following a high-protein diet to support muscle growth, recovery, satiety, and energy. Balancing this with a low-FODMAP diet may seem overwhelming at first. Nevertheless, achieving this balance is possible with careful planning and a few resourceful recipes.

Protein isn't just essential; it's crucial for those leading an active lifestyle. It is the primary building block for muscle growth and repair, particularly during strength training. Consuming protein-rich foods after exercise is not only beneficial but necessary. It helps reduce muscle soreness, encourages muscle protein synthesis, and enhances recovery. Protein also provides a feeling of fullness and satisfaction, preventing overeating and aiding in weight management. Additionally, it serves as an alternative energy source when carbohydrate and fat stores are low.

Protein should comprise around 10-35% of daily caloric intake for active adults. However, this can vary depending on factors such as age, sex, weight, and level of physical activity, with those engaging in more intense or prolonged exercise potentially requiring more protein. Obtaining sufficient protein can be challenging on a low-FODMAP diet, as some common high-protein foods may be high in FODMAPs. Nonetheless, careful planning and food selection can effectively meet these protein needs.

Within a low-FODMAP diet, you can enjoy various protein-rich foods. Animal-based proteins, such as eggs and lactose-free dairy products, including lactose-free milk, hard cheeses, and lactose-free yogurts, are excellent protein sources and provide essential nutrients like calcium and vitamin D. Plant-based proteins like firm tofu and tempeh, as well as some nuts and seeds, including walnuts, macadamia nuts, and chia seeds, are low in FODMAPs and offer decent protein content. Some low-FODMAP grains, like quinoa and brown rice, are reliable sources of plant-based protein, with quinoa being a complete protein that contains all the essential amino acids the body needs. With such a diverse range of options, you can feel confident in meeting your protein needs while managing your IBS symptoms.

When maintaining a balanced, low-FODMAP, high-protein diet, it's essential to include a source of protein in every meal or snack. Additionally, it must contain carbohydrates for energy, healthy fats for nutrient absorption and satiety, and a variety of low-FODMAP vegetables for volume, fiber, and essential nutrients.

Adjusting portion sizes according to your body's hunger and fullness cues is crucial to maintaining a balanced diet. Remember to be mindful of this. Planning meals and snacks ahead of time can help ensure they are balanced and alleviate the stress of deciding what to eat. Everyone's needs differ, and eating in a way that feels best for you is essential.

Pre- and post-workout nutrition is essential for those combining a low-FODMAP diet with a high-protein diet. The meals or snacks consumed before and after workouts should be accessible on the stomach yet provide the necessary nutrients for physical activity.

Navigating the balance between low-FODMAP and high-protein diets for an active lifestyle can seem challenging. However, you can manage IBS symptoms while meeting your nutritional needs by understanding how these dietary needs intersect and arming yourself with intelligent strategies and creative recipes. The key lies in meticulous planning, mindful food selections, well-rounded meals, and adaptability. Always remember managing IBS symptoms and enjoying a healthy, active lifestyle are not mutually exclusive goals. You can enjoy the best of both worlds by effectively combining a low-FODMAP diet with a high-protein diet.

COMMON CONCERNS ABOUT THE LOW-FODMAP DIET

The low FODMAP diet is an effective strategy for managing irritable bowel syndrome (IBS). Still, it can sometimes raise some concerns for people who intend to follow this approach, such as the impact this diet may have on social life, the confusion generated by often conflicting information, and, last but not least, the harsh dietary restrictions required.

Below are some valuable tips that can help you overcome these concerns.

First, managing social life and food events (such as lunches or dinners out at friends' or restaurants) can be addressed, for example, by checking the restaurant menu in advance (on the website or on some of the most popular apps that collect customer reviews), asking about the ingredients used in the preparation of the dishes you intend to eat, or simply communicating (to the waiter or friends) your dietary needs.

Despite often discordant information about the low-FODMAP diet, in today's digital age, it is crucial to rely on reliable sources and stay informed about the latest research. In this regard, the best thing to do is rely on studies conducted by Monash University.

Finally, the previous chapters specifically addressed the issue of restricting the intake of certain types of foods to gain benefits on the manifestation of symptoms of IBS and other digestive disorders. Nonetheless, anyone wishing to tackle this diet can identify alternative food sources that provide nutritional and caloric intake while being low in FODMAPs. In all cases, people can locate food alternatives, even if they adopt a vegetarian lifestyle or suffer from food intolerances.

It is essential to specify and remember that the restrictions required by the low FODMAP diet are confined mainly to the initial phase of the diet, i.e., the elimination phase.

In conclusion, the low FODMAP diet is an effective tool for those suffering from gastrointestinal disorders and versatile in that it can perfectly mold itself to any lifestyle. For this reason, a healthy understanding of this approach can help you not only face without anxiety the social events in which you participate but also increase your social life and live it to the fullest with satisfaction.

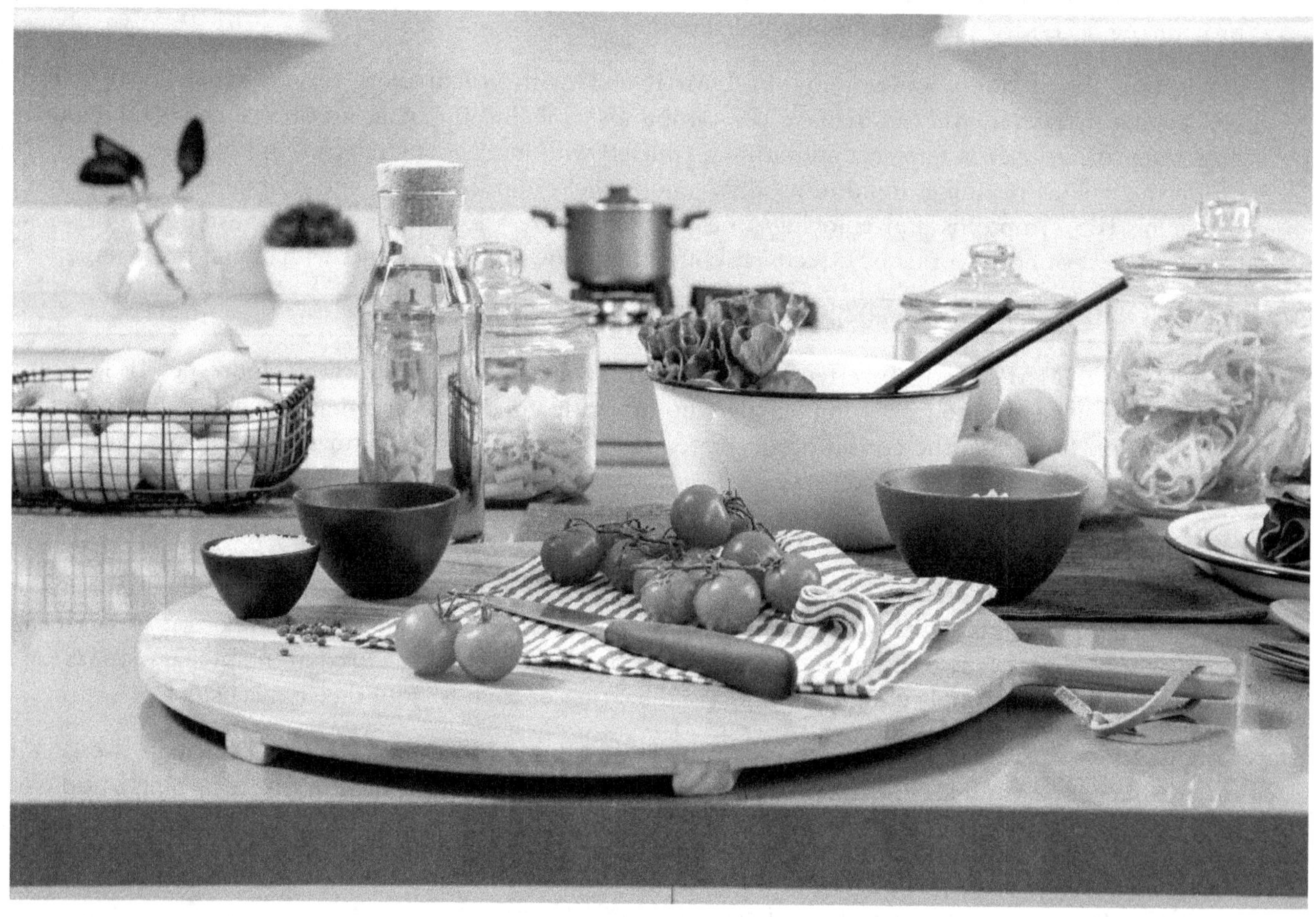

Embarking on the low-FODMAP diet journey requires a well-organized kitchen layout. A well-prepared kitchen can significantly contribute to your success with the diet, making it easier to stick to the recommended food choices. This guide outlines the steps to declutter, organize, and stock your kitchen successfully. It also offers tips for grocery shopping and meal prepping, helping create a streamlined environment conducive to your low-FODMAP diet.

Take pride in the first step of your journey-decluttering your kitchen. This process will help you eliminate high-FODMAP foods and reduce the temptation that could derail your diet plan. Start by examining every item in your pantry, fridge, and freezer, identifying those high in FODMAPs. Once you have categorized your food into high-FODMAP, low-FODMAP, and uncertain categories, decide how to dispose of high-FODMAP foods. If unopened, consider donating them to a local food bank or giving them to family or friends. Remember to dispose of opened items that cannot be donated to remove temptation. Lastly, arrange your low-FODMAP foods for easy access and research any items you need clarification on.

Empower yourself by understanding what constitutes low-FODMAP foods. This knowledge is critical to effectively stocking your kitchen. Familiarize yourself with low-FODMAP food options, which span all food groups and offer a variety of choices. Learning to read food labels for high-FODMAP ingredients is crucial, and using reliable tools, like the Monash University FODMAP app, can facilitate this process.

After decluttering your kitchen and becoming familiar with low-FODMAP foods, you can restock your pantry, fridge, and freezer. Having a variety of available foods facilitates meal preparation and adherence to your diet. Your pantry should include grains like rice, quinoa, gluten-free pasta, canned goods, herbs, spices, and oils. At the same time, your fridge should contain:

- Fresh low-FODMAP fruits and vegetables
- Lactose-free dairy or alternatives
- Fresh proteins

Freezer essentials include low-FODMAP vegetables and fruits, homemade meals, gluten-free bread, and frozen proteins. Remember to stock up on low-FODMAP-friendly drinks and ready-to-eat snacks.

Categorizing your foods is a practical approach to organizing your kitchen and meal planning. Using clear containers for storage and keeping a separate space for high-FODMAP foods if you live with others who are not following the diet will also help avoid confusion.

Smart grocery shopping is integral to maintaining your low-FODMAP diet. Plan your meals, create a shopping list, and learn to navigate the supermarket, focusing on the fresh food sections typically found around the perimeter. Label reading skills are essential here, too. Even in this case, The Monash University FODMAP app is a valuable tool to help you identify high-FODMAP ingredients and make informed food choices. Be cautious with 'Free From' foods, as they may not necessarily be low-FODMAP, and plan for snacks to prevent hunger and potential diet deviations.

It's essential to prioritize meal preparation and planning, especially for those with busy schedules. This involves scheduling your weekly meals, creating a meal prep plan, and utilizing batch cooking to save time. Batch cooking includes making large portions of food and dividing them for later use. This method can help you save time and energy throughout the week and ensure you always have a low-FODMAP meal available. To effectively batch cook, opt for recipes that can be easily scaled up, invest in high-quality storage containers, and consider using a slow cooker or pressure cooker to save even more time.

Lastly, equip your kitchen with essential tools to make your Low-FODMAP cooking experience more efficient and enjoyable. Essential tools include excellent knives for chopping fruits and vegetables, cutting boards for food preparation, measuring cups and spoons for accurate portioning, mixing bowls for combining ingredients, pots and pans for cooking, utensils for stirring and serving, a colander for draining pasta and vegetables, kitchen appliances like a blender or food processor for making sauces and smoothies, and storage containers for keeping your food fresh. Investing in food prep tools like a vegetable peeler, mandoline slicer, box grater, garlic press, and kitchen scale can simplify the process. For storage, consider using airtight containers, produce saver containers, freezer bags, pantry organizers, mason jars, a label maker, lunch containers, and spice jars. Although not essential, additional extras may prove beneficial depending on your cooking habits.

Preparing your kitchen for the low-FODMAP diet will create a supportive environment to facilitate your dietary transition, making it easier to manage your symptoms and enjoy various delicious, nutritious meals.

GROCERY SHOPPING GUIDE FOR LOW-FODMAP FOODS

Keeping a low-FODMAP diet while grocery shopping can feel overwhelming as you must avoid certain foods and ingredients. However, with proper preparation and understanding, shopping for low-FODMAP foods can be more accessible and enjoyable. It's crucial to have a flexible plan that saves time, reduces stress, and prevents accidental purchases of high-FODMAP foods. This includes creating a shopping list, researching low-FODMAP products online, and preparing snacks and quick meals for unexpected hunger or busy days.

Knowing the layout of your grocery store will help you efficiently shop for low-FODMAP items. Focus on the perimeter for fresh produce, meat, and dairy, but also be aware of essential low-FODMAP items in the middle aisles. Look for cheaper options on higher and lower shelves and make the most of the bulk section. Eating before you shop can prevent impulse buying and be ready to visit multiple stores to find all your low-FODMAP foods.

Empower yourself by reading food labels carefully. Check ingredients, pay attention to their order, and watch out for high-FODMAP ingredients like fructose, lactose, fructans, galactans, and polyols. Be wary of hidden FODMAPs in products like onion powder, wheat, or high-fructose corn syrup. Consider using FODMAP apps to help identify high and low-FODMAP foods.

When buying fresh produce, familiarize yourself with low-FODMAP fruits and vegetables and choose fresh produce over packaged ones. Seasonal produce is often cheaper and fresher, and knowing how to spot freshness can be helpful. Pay attention to serving sizes and prepare your produce when you get home.

Make sure to include a balance of grains, proteins, and dairy in your diet. Opt for low-FODMAP grains, unprocessed meats and fish, specific cheeses, and lactose-free yogurts. Always be mindful of hidden FODMAPs and find alternatives for common high-FODMAP foods.

Having low-FODMAP pantry staples and a selection of snacks is essential to maintain steady energy levels. If you enjoy baking, stock up on low-FODMAP baking ingredients. Keeping quick low-FODMAP meals in your pantry is advisable for busy days.

The journey of the low-FODMAP diet may present challenges, such as a limited selection of low-FODMAP foods, accommodating other diets when cooking, unplanned grocery store trips, or accidentally purchasing high-FODMAP foods. However, people can typically overcome these challenges. The low-FODMAP diet can remain manageable, effective, and enjoyable by devising strategies to manage these obstacles. Effective grocery shopping for a low-FODMAP diet requires proper planning, a keen understanding of food labels, and adaptability to overcome potential setbacks and challenges.

A low-FODMAP diet is central to managing irritable bowel syndrome (IBS), a long-term commitment that requires an integrated plan. This plan should consider individual triggers, dietary restrictions, and lifestyle modifications. Creating a low-FODMAP meal plan that suits your weekly schedule and nutritional preferences can prevent impulse eating and ensure consistent access to low-FODMAP meals, effectively managing IBS symptoms.

Time-saving strategies such as batch cooking, meal prepping in advance, and using leftovers can simplify the cooking process. It's essential to prepare for social situations and dining out in advance, which can be done through effective communication and occasional flexibility.

It's crucial to remember that managing IBS goes beyond short-term diet changes and requires sustainable strategies that consider your unique triggers, lifestyle, and nutritional needs. Therefore, devising a long-term plan is not just beneficial; it's a source of relief and comfort. It provides sustained symptom relief, adapts to changes in your body's response to different foods, allows for personalized modifications, ensures balanced nutrition, and improves overall quality of life.

Personalizing your diet is crucial to your long-term plan. This can be achieved by identifying your triggers, creating a personalized food list, and considering your lifestyle and preferences. Ensuring balanced nutrition is also crucial. Regularly monitoring and making necessary adjustments based on your body's responses play an essential role in maintaining your diet, making it uniquely your plan.

Lifestyle changes are crucial for effective IBS management, in addition to dietary modifications. Regular physical activity, stress management techniques, adequate sleep, and proper hydration can significantly influence your IBS symptoms. But remember, you're not alone in this journey. Regular medical check-ups and professional guidance are also beneficial for monitoring your condition, discussing your diet plan, and providing the emotional support you need.

Remember, a balanced diet and a healthy lifestyle are not just about managing IBS symptoms; they're vital for overall health. A balanced Low-FODMAP diet ensures you get all the nutrients your body needs, including a balance of macronutrients and micronutrients, plenty of low-FODMAP fruits and vegetables, and adequate hydration. Regular physical activity, quality sleep, stress management, and routine medical check-ups contribute to a healthier lifestyle, benefiting you beyond IBS management.

In conclusion, managing IBS symptoms requires a holistic approach encompassing a low-FODMAP diet, personalized long-term plans, regular monitoring, lifestyle modifications, and professional guidance. By following these strategies, you can lead a fulfilling life without letting IBS define you.

Navigating the complexities of social life while adhering to a low-FODMAP diet can be challenging. However, you can overcome these challenges with thoughtful strategies, effective communication, and a flexible approach.

Recognizing the Importance of Communication

Communication forms the cornerstone of successfully maintaining your social life while following a low-FODMAP diet. It is crucial to convey your dietary needs to friends, family, and hosts. If you are dining out, discussing your nutritional requirements with the server or chef is often crucial to having a meal that aligns with your diet. Remember, most people are understanding and accommodating when aware of your needs.

The Role of Planning

Planning can significantly alleviate the anxiety associated with social events or dinner parties. If you are invited to a social gathering, find out about the menu in advance and consider bringing a Low-FODMAP dish to share. When dining out, reviewing the restaurant's menu online can help you identify suitable options.

Embracing Flexibility

It is essential to focus on dietary possibilities rather than limitations. You can usually find something suitable on the menu—like grilled meat or fish with vegetables or a salad without onions, garlic, or high-FODMAP dressings. Creativity and flexibility are paramount in successfully incorporating a low-FODMAP diet into a vibrant social life.

The Value of Being Prepared

Having Low-FODMAP snacks readily available can be a lifesaver if there are no suitable food options at a social event. Consider carrying a small bag of nuts, a piece of fruit, or a homemade Low-FODMAP snack bar when you are out.

Educating Yourself and Others

The more knowledgeable you are about your diet, the easier it will be to navigate social situations. Learning about suitable food and drink options, understanding that portion size can affect FODMAP levels, and sharing this information with others can help create a supportive environment for managing your diet.

Staying Socially Active

Maintaining your social life is crucial while managing your diet. If a social event is causing anxiety, consider discussing your worries with a trusted friend, family member, or dietitian. They can provide guidance and reassurance and offer new strategies for managing social situations.

Practicing Self-Care

Embarking on a new diet can be stressful, especially when navigating social situations. Remember to prioritize your mental health and consider seeking support from a mental health professional if needed. Coping mechanisms such as deep-breathing exercises or meditation can help manage diet-related stress.

A Future of Dietary Flexibility

The low-FODMAP diet is not often a lifelong commitment. After the elimination phase, you will gradually reintroduce foods to identify triggers, making your diet less restrictive. Remember this when dining out or attending social events, as this can alleviate some of the pressure associated with adhering strictly to your diet.

Putting It All Together

Adhering to a low-FODMAP diet while maintaining an active social life requires a delicate balance of communication, planning, flexibility, and education. Whether dining out, attending a party, or traveling, remember to prioritize your dietary needs without isolating yourself. Having supportive people around you, practicing self-care, and keeping the future of your diet in perspective can all contribute to successfully managing social situations. While the process may require additional effort and adjustments, remember that your well-being and enjoyment are the goal. With these strategies, you can continue to savor your social life while managing your IBS symptoms effectively.

HANDLING MISINFORMATION ABOUT THE LOW-FODMAP DIET

In today's digital era, an excess of information is available, making it essential to distinguish facts from fiction, especially regarding diet trends like the Low-FODMAP diet. This diet aims to alleviate the symptoms of Irritable Bowel Syndrome (IBS) and has become popular. However, misinformation has also spread along with its popularity. Recognizing this problem is crucial to successfully following an effective low-FODMAP diet. This discussion aims to provide strategies and resources for dealing with such misinformation.

Various sources could present misinformation about the low-FODMAP diet, such as providing overly simplistic explanations like 'all high-FODMAP foods are bad ', overgeneralizations such as 'everyone with IBS should follow this diet ', absolutes like 'this diet will cure your IBS ', quick fixes or miraculous claims. These can be misleading and result in an inaccurate understanding of the diet. Please remember to cautiously approach information that needs more credible sources or is backed by non-expert opinions. It's crucial to remember that the low-FODMAP diet is a complex dietary approach that requires personalization. While it can be highly effective, it is not a miracle cure or a one-size-fits-all solution.

Familiar sources of misinformation include:

- Social media.
- Non-expert blogs.
- Misinterpreted scientific studies.
- Well-meaning friends and family.
- Fad diet books or programs.

While these platforms can provide helpful tips and shared experiences, they may also promote misleading or inaccurate information about the low-FODMAP diet. Following such misinformation can lead to ineffective management of IBS symptoms, unnecessary dietary restrictions, or even health risks. Therefore, it is essential to critically evaluate the information and consider its source before making dietary decisions.

Evaluating information about the low-FODMAP diet requires critical thinking skills. Remember to consider the source of information, look for evidence supporting the claims, check when the data was last updated, beware of sensationalism, consult multiple sources, and trust your instincts. However, the best source of advice about your diet will always be a healthcare provider who knows your health history and needs. It's crucial to consult them before making significant dietary changes, especially if you have a medical condition like IBS.

It is also important to dispel common myths about the low-FODMAP diet, such as that it is gluten-free, a lifetime diet, or that it will lead to weight loss. Clearing these misconceptions can set realistic expectations and lead to a more successful diet implementation.

Relying on credible sources can help you understand the low-FODMAP diet accurately. Registered dietitians, gastroenterologists, reputable health organizations, Monash University, peer-reviewed journals, and IBS support groups are all reliable sources of information. These resources can provide accurate, up-to-date, and evidence-based information about the low-FODMAP diet.

Your personal experience is a powerful tool when following the low-FODMAP diet. Individual responses to the diet vary, and understanding your body's reactions to different foods is critical to tailor the diet to your needs. This personal understanding, scientific evidence, and expert advice empower you to navigate a successful and sustainable low-FODMAP diet.

Armed with accurate knowledge, you have the opportunity to contribute to the understanding of the low-FODMAP diet. Whether by educating your social circle, sharing reliable sources, advocating in social situations, sharing your personal experience, or supporting others on the same journey, your actions can make it easier for others to find effective strategies for managing their IBS symptoms. Your role in spreading accurate information is crucial and can make a significant difference.

In conclusion, while navigating the sea of misinformation about the low-FODMAP diet can be challenging, it's important to remember that when understood and personalized, this diet can be a highly effective strategy for managing IBS symptoms. By developing a critical eye, relying on reliable resources, learning from individual experiences, and spreading accurate information, you can successfully manage your IBS symptoms while helping others on the same journey. A combined effort of science and unique understanding makes the Low-FODMAP diet a successful strategy for many dealing with IBS.

UNDERSTANDING AND LISTENING TO YOUR BODY'S RESPONSES

Mastering the art of managing Irritable Bowel Syndrome (IBS) through diet is a journey that begins with a heightened sense of awareness about your body's responses. This is what we call interoception or body awareness, and it's not just a fancy term- it's a powerful tool that can help you understand and identify the internal cues and signals sent by your body. These signals can be as subtle as a feeling of hunger or fullness or as noticeable as physical discomfort or minor changes in bowel habits.

The importance of body awareness in managing IBS is multifold:

1. It aids in identifying and recognizing symptoms associated with IBS. This early detection can assist in initiative-taking IBS management.
2. It helps understand your unique food triggers by observing your body's reaction to several types of food.
3. It allows you to identify your stress signals, which can help manage stress-triggered IBS episodes.
4. It can enhance communication with healthcare providers as you can provide accurate information about your symptoms and reactions.
5. Body awareness leads to personal empowerment, allowing you to take control of your IBS management.

Recognizing your body's signs and symptoms is vital for managing IBS. Since IBS symptoms can vary significantly between individuals, understanding your unique signs and symptoms allows you to mitigate them effectively. Symptoms may include common IBS symptoms such as abdominal pain, bloating, altered bowel habits, and less common ones like nausea, fatigue, backache, and urinary problems. Identifying when your symptoms occur and observing their severity is critical to understanding your body's responses to potential triggers.

One of the most effective ways to gain control over your IBS symptoms is by maintaining a food and symptom diary. This simple yet powerful tool can help you track your symptoms and food intake, allowing you to see patterns and correlations that might otherwise go unnoticed. By recording all foods and drinks consumed, along with additional factors like stress, physical activity, sleep, and medication, you can build a comprehensive picture of your IBS management. Regular diary reviews can be a game-changer, helping you identify triggers and make informed dietary adjustments.

Understanding your body's response to FODMAPs is crucial to personalizing your low-FODMAP diet and gaining better control over your IBS symptoms. Immediate versus delayed reactions, the severity of reactions, individual differences in tolerance, and the role of stress and other factors all play a part in your body's response to FODMAPs.

Mindfulness is a powerful tool that can enhance body awareness, helping you become more attuned to your body's signals. It's not just about managing symptoms; it's about reducing stress and finding a sense of calm amidst the challenges of IBS.

Interpreting body signals is critical in personalizing your diet for IBS management. By identifying trigger foods, considering the amount consumed, testing and retesting foods, making gradual dietary changes, maintaining nutritional balance, staying flexible, and consulting a healthcare professional, when necessary, you can make informed dietary adjustments that help manage your symptoms effectively.

In conclusion, understanding and responding to your body's signals is a journey. It's an ongoing process that requires patience and careful observation. But remember, you're not alone in this. With the right tools and support, it can lead to an improved quality of life.

What are FODMAPs?

FERMENTABLE

OLIGOSACCHARIDES

DISACCHARIDES

MONOSACCHARIDES

AND

POLYOLS

Understanding the nuances of FODMAP levels in foods is crucial for effectively managing IBS symptoms. The low-FODMAP diet doesn't require eliminating certain foods but rather moderation and balance based on individual tolerance. Paying attention to serving sizes is vital in this context. Even foods low in FODMAPs can trigger symptoms if consumed excessively. On the other hand, small amounts of certain high-FODMAP foods may be tolerated. This underscores the significance of understanding FODMAP stacking – the cumulative impact of consuming various low-FODMAP foods together, leading to a high overall FODMAP intake. For instance, if you consume a large portion of low-FODMAP food and then drink another low-FODMAP food, the total FODMAP content of your meal may be high. This can lead to symptoms, even if each food individually is low in FODMAPs. A food diary can help understand personal tolerance and establish suitable portion sizes. Seeking professional guidance from a dietitian can further assist in clarifying appropriate serving sizes and understanding the potential implications of FODMAP stacking.

Reading food labels is a crucial step in managing FODMAP intake. Many processed and packaged foods contain hidden FODMAPs in their ingredients. To decode food labels, start by looking for high-FODMAP ingredients such as honey, high fructose corn syrup, inulin, wheat, rye, lactose, and ingredients ending in "-ol" (like sorbitol, mannitol, and xylitol). Understanding the listing order of components can also provide insight into the quantity of potential high-FODMAP elements in the product. For example, if a high-FODMAP ingredient is listed first, it means the product contains a significant amount of it. While labels like 'suitable for vegans' or 'gluten-free' can be helpful, they do not necessarily mean the product is low in FODMAPs. Tools such as Low-FODMAP certification logos and FODMAP-specific apps can aid in navigating the maze of food labels.

Understanding FODMAPs is a journey that is continually evolving; it is essential to stay updated and adapt to these changes. Regular knowledge updates, using trusted resources, maintaining flexibility in dietary choices, collaborating with a dietitian, and participating in the FODMAP community can be beneficial in staying abreast of the latest developments in the world of FODMAPs. This active engagement with the latest research can make you feel informed and proactive in managing your IBS symptoms.

Effectively navigating low, medium, and high-FODMAP foods involves:

- A comprehensive understanding of food content.
- A mindful approach to portion sizes.
- The ability to decode food labels.
- A commitment to staying updated with current research.

It's a delicate balance to strike, but with the proper knowledge, practice, and guidance, individuals with IBS can effectively manage their symptoms and maintain a varied, enjoyable diet. This reassurance is to instill a sense of hope and confidence in your ability to manage your IBS symptoms. You have the power to take control of your health and live a fulfilling life despite your IBS.

Low-FODMAP foods contain insignificant amounts of FODMAPs and are typically well-tolerated by individuals with IBS. These foods can form the basis of your diet during the elimination phase and beyond. Here are some examples of low-FODMAP foods, categorized by food group:

Fruits: Certain fruits are low in FODMAPs and can be enjoyed freely. These include bananas, oranges, grapes, strawberries, blueberries, kiwi, pineapple, and papaya.

Vegetables: Many vegetables are low in FODMAPs. Examples include carrots, bell peppers, cucumbers, lettuce, tomatoes, zucchini, eggplant, potatoes, and green beans.

Grains: Several grains and cereals are low in FODMAPs. These include rice, oats, quinoa, cornmeal, and gluten-free flour (like rice flour or corn flour).

Proteins: Most proteins are low in FODMAPs; This includes meat, fish, chicken, tofu, tempeh, and certain nuts and seeds (like walnuts and pumpkin seeds).

Dairy Products: Lactose-free dairy products are low in FODMAPs. These include lactose-free milk, hard cheeses, and certain types of yogurts. Plant-based milks like almond and rice milk are also typically low in FODMAPs.

Sweeteners: Certain sweeteners are low in FODMAPs. These include maple syrup, table sugar (sucrose), and certain artificial sweeteners (aspartame and sucralose).

Beverages: Many beverages, including water, coffee, most teas, and certain fruit juices (like cranberry juice), are low in FODMAPs.

It's important to remember that even with low-FODMAP foods, portion sizes matter. Overconsumption could potentially trigger symptoms. So, while these foods are generally well-tolerated, it's crucial to be mindful of how much you're eating. Everyone is unique, and what works for one person may not work for another. So, as always, listening to your body and making individualized dietary adjustments is key.

LOW FODMAP FOOD LIST

OLIGOSACCHARIDES	
Fruits	Bananas (not overripe), Oranges, Pineapples, Strawberries, Blueberries, Grapes, Kiwi
Vegetables	Bell peppers, Carrots, Cucumbers, Eggplant, Lettuce, Tomatoes, Bamboo shoots, Bok choy, Zucchini
Grains	Quinoa, Rice (all types), Oats, Gluten-free pasta, Corn (including popcorn), Sorghum
Dairy	dairy products typically do not contain Oligosaccharides
Nuts and Seeds	nuts & seeds typically do not contain Oligosaccharides

DISACCHARIDES	
Fruits	Fruits typically do not contain Disaccharides
Vegetables	Vegetables typically do not contain Disaccharides
Grains	Grains typically do not contain Disaccharides
Dairy	Lactose-free milk, Lactose-free yogurt, Lactose-free cottage cheese, Hard cheeses (like cheddar, parmesan, Swiss, Pecorino), Butter
Nuts and Seeds	nuts & seeds typically do not contain Disaccharides

MONOSACCHARIDES	
Fruits	Kiwi, Lemons, Limes, Papaya, Passionfruit, Banana, Blueberries, Strawberries, Orange Grapes, Pineapple
Vegetables	Alfalfa, Bamboo shoots, Bok choy, Green beans, Kale, Carrots, Bell Peppers, Cucumber, Lettuce, Tomato, Zucchini, Spinach
Grains	Millet, Oats, Quinoa, Rice, Sorghum, Rice, Corn
Dairy	Dairy typically do not contain Monosaccharides
Nuts and Seeds	Almonds (in small quantities), Hazelnuts, Pecans, Poppy seeds, Walnuts, Pine nuts, Sunflower seeds, Pumpkin seeds

POLYOLS	
Fruits	Bananas, Blueberries, Kiwi, Oranges, Pineapple, Grapes, Strawberries
Vegetables	Bell peppers, Carrots, Lettuce, Parsnip, Tomato, Cucumbers, Zucchini, Spinach
Grains	Gluten-free bread, Quinoa, Rice, Sourdough spelt, Oats, Corn
Dairy	Dairy typically do not contain Polyols
Nuts and Seeds	Nuts and Seeds typically do not contain Polyols

High-FODMAP foods, which are common in many people's diets, contain significant amounts of fermentable carbohydrates that can trigger symptoms in individuals with IBS. These foods are diverse, spanning various categories, including fruits, vegetables, grains, proteins, dairy products, and sweeteners. Here is a non-exhaustive list of common high-FODMAP foods within these categories:

Fruits: Certain fruits are high in FODMAPs, especially those containing excess fructose. These include apples, pears, mangoes, cherries, peaches, plums, and watermelon. Dried fruits and fruit juices are high in FODMAPs as well.

Vegetables: Some vegetables high in FODMAPs include onions, garlic, asparagus, artichokes, peas, mushrooms, cauliflower, and beetroot.

Grains: Certain grains and cereals are high in FODMAPs. These include wheat and rye in substantial amounts, such as in bread, pasta, and cereals. Barley is also a high-FODMAP grain.

Proteins: While most proteins are not a source of FODMAPs, certain types, such as legumes (e.g., chickpeas, lentils, and beans) and some nuts and seeds, can be high in FODMAPs.

Dairy Products: Lactose-containing dairy products are high in FODMAPs. These include milk (from cows, goats, and sheep), soft cheese, yogurt, and ice cream.

Sweeteners: Sweeteners can be a significant source of FODMAPs. Honey and high fructose corn syrup are high in FODMAPs, as are sweeteners ending in "-ol," such as sorbitol, mannitol, and xylitol.

Processed Foods: Processed foods can often contain hidden FODMAPs. Look for high-FODMAP ingredients such as inulin, wheat flour, high fructose corn syrup, and particular fruit and vegetable juices or concentrates.

Remember, there are plenty of low-FODMAP alternatives available for many of these high-FODMAP foods. FODMAP tolerance can vary among individuals. Some people may be able to consume lesser amounts of these foods without experiencing symptoms, while others may be more sensitive. It is also important to note that many of these foods have low-FODMAP alternatives and can be reintroduced into the diet during maintenance to identify personal tolerances.

HIGH FODMAP FOOD LIST

OLIGOSACCHARIDES	
Fruits	Raspberries, Blackberries, Pomegranates, Tamarillos, Apples, Mango, Rambutan, Watermelon, Nectarines, Pears, White Peaches
Vegetables	Artichokes, Asparagus, Broccoli, Garlic, Onions, Leek bulb, Beetroot, Savoy Cabbage
Grains	Rye, Barley, Spelt, Inulin, Wheat (in substantial amounts)
Dairy	Oligosaccharides are not found in dairy products
Nuts and Seeds	Cashews, Pistachios, Soybeans, Chickpeas

DISACCHARIDES	
Fruits	Disaccharides such as lactose are not found in fruits
Vegetables	Disaccharides such as lactose are not found in vegetables
Grains	Disaccharides such as lactose are not found in grains
Dairy	Milk (cow, goat, and sheep), Yogurt, Ice cream, Soft cheeses like Ricotta and Cottage cheese, Custard
Nuts and Seeds	Disaccharides such as lactose are not found in nuts and seeds

MONOSACCHARIDES	
Fruits	Apples, Pears, Watermelon, Mangoes, Cherries, High-fructose dried fruits (like dates, prunes and raisins)
Vegetables	Asparagus, Sugar snap peas, Artichokes, Onions (all types)
Grains	Wheat, Rye, Raisins, corn syrup
Dairy	Dairy products do not usually contain prominent levels of fructose.
Nuts and Seeds	Nuts and seeds do not typically contain prominent levels of fructose

POLYOLS	
Fruits	Apples, Apricots, Blackberries, Cherries, Peaches, Avocados, Nectarines, Pears, Plums, Prunes, Watermelon
Vegetables	Cauliflower, Mushrooms, Snow peas
Grains	Wheat-based products
Dairy	Dairy products do not usually contain prominent levels of polyols
Nuts and Seeds	Some nut and seed varieties can have added polyols, especially those labelled as "sugar-free" or "no added sugar"

BREAKFAST RECIPES

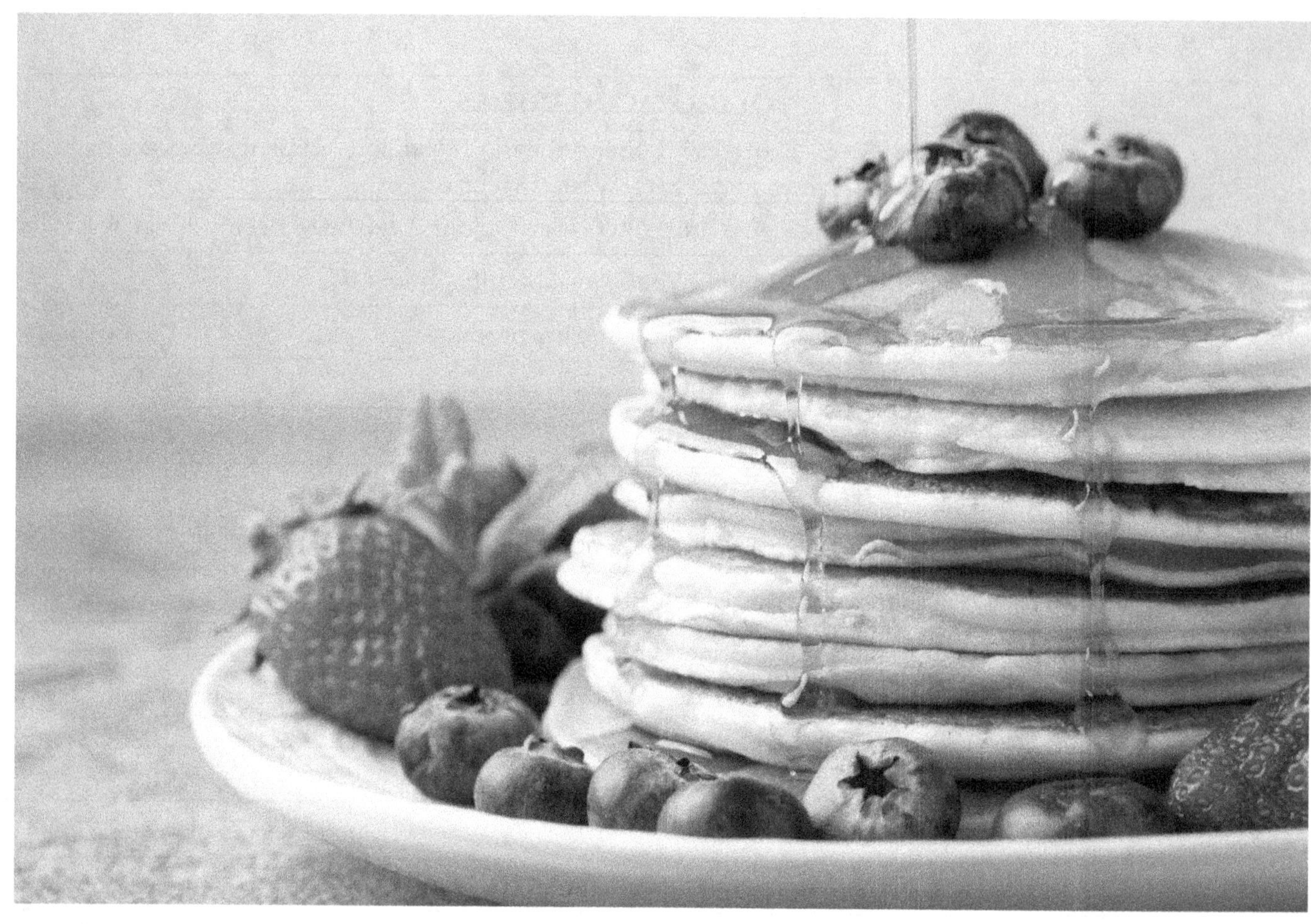

1. QUICK AND EASY BANANA PANCAKES (V)

Preparation Time: 10 minutes | Cooking Time: 15 minutes | Serves: 2

Ingredients:

- 2 ripe bananas
- 2 large eggs
- 1/2 cup of gluten-free oats
- 1/4 teaspoon of cinnamon
- 1/2 teaspoon of baking powder
- A pinch of salt
- 1/2 teaspoon of pure vanilla extract (optional)
- Non-dairy milk as needed (e.g., almond milk, but only if the batter is too thick)
- A small amount of olive oil for cooking

Instructions:

1. In a blender, combine the bananas, eggs, oats, cinnamon, baking powder, salt, and vanilla extract. Blend until smooth.
2. If the batter seems too thick, add a small amount of non-dairy milk and blend again.
3. Heat a non-stick skillet over medium heat and lightly coat with olive oil.
4. Pour a small amount of batter onto the skillet for each pancake. Cook for 2-3 minutes on each side or until golden brown.
5. Repeat with the remaining batter.
6. Serve the pancakes warm. You can top them with a small amount of maple syrup if desired or enjoy as they are.

Nutritional Values: Calories: 260 | Protein: 9g | Carbohydrates: 45g | Fiber: 5g | Sugar: 20g | Fat: 6g

2. SPINACH AND FETA FRITTATA

Preparation Time: 10 minutes | Cooking Time: 20 minutes | Serves: 4

Ingredients:

- 8 large eggs
- 1/4 cup lactose-free milk
- 1/2 teaspoon salt
- 1/4 teaspoon black pepper
- 1 tablespoon garlic-infused olive oil
- 2 cups fresh spinach
- 1/2 cup feta cheese (ensure it is low in lactose)

Instructions:

1. Preheat your oven to 350°F (175°C).
2. In a large bowl, whisk together the eggs, lactose-free milk, salt, and pepper. Set aside.
3. Heat the garlic-infused olive oil in a 10-inch oven-safe skillet over medium heat. Add the spinach and sauté until wilted, about 2-3 minutes.

Spread the wilted spinach evenly across the skillet. Pour the egg mixture over the spinach.

4. Sprinkle the feta cheese evenly over the top of the egg mixture.
5. Place the skillet in the preheated oven and bake for 15-20 minutes, or until the frittata is set and lightly golden on top.
6. Allow the frittata to cool for a few minutes before slicing and serving.

Nutritional Values: Calories: 230 | Protein: 16g | Carbohydrates: 3g | Fiber: 1g | Sugar: 2g | Fat: 17g

Note: Ensure your feta cheese is low in lactose. If you are unsure, lactose-free versions are available.

3. Low-FODMAP Friendly Smoothie Bowl (V)

Preparation Time: 10 minutes | Cooking Time: 0 minutes | Serves: 1

Ingredients:

- 1 ripe banana
- 1/2 cup frozen strawberries
- 1/2 cup lactose-free yogurt or almond milk yogurt
- 1 tablespoon chia seeds
- 1 tablespoon peanut butter
- Optional toppings: a small handful of blueberries, sliced kiwi (both are low FODMAP fruits)

Instructions:

1. In a blender, combine the banana, strawberries, yogurt or almond milk yogurt, chia seeds, and peanut butter.
2. Blend until smooth and creamy. If the mixture is too thick, you can add a small amount of water or additional yogurt to reach your desired consistency.
3. Pour the smoothie into a bowl.
4. Arrange your chosen toppings on the smoothie in an appealing pattern.
5. Enjoy your smoothie bowl immediately, as the mixture can thicken if left to sit.

Nutritional Values: Calories: 390 | Protein: 14g | Carbohydrates: 58g | Fiber: 13g | Sugar: 30g | Fat: 15g

Note: Almond milk yogurt and peanut butter are low FODMAP, but brands can vary. If you have a nut allergy, you can substitute sunflower seed butter for the peanut butter.

4. Overnight Chia Pudding with Berries (VG)

Preparation Time: 10 minutes | Resting Time: 8 hours | Serves: 2

Ingredients:

- 1/4 cup chia seeds
- 1 cup almond milk or another non-dairy milk
- 1 tablespoon pure maple syrup
- 1/2 teaspoon pure vanilla extract
- 1 cup mixed berries (strawberries, blueberries, and kiwi)

Instructions:

1. In a bowl or jar, combine the chia seeds, almond milk, maple syrup, and vanilla extract.
2. Stir well to make sure the chia seeds are evenly distributed.
3. Cover and refrigerate overnight (or at least for 6 hours).
4. In the morning, give the chia pudding a good stir to break up any clumps.
5. Top the chia pudding with the mixed berries before serving.

Nutritional Values: Calories: 220 | Protein: 6g | Carbohydrates: 29g | Fiber: 12g | Sugar: 14g | Fat: 9g

Note: Most non-dairy milks are low FODMAP, but brands can vary. If you have a nut allergy, you can substitute oat milk or rice milk for the almond milk. As a sweetener, we use maple syrup, but you can use another low FODMAP sweetener if preferred.

Preparation Time: 5 minutes | Cooking Time: 10 minutes | Serves: 1

Ingredients:

- 2 large eggs
- Salt and pepper to taste
- 1 tablespoon garlic-infused olive oil
- 1 gluten-free tortilla wrap
- 1/4 cup shredded cheddar cheese (lactose-free if needed)
- 1 handful of spinach leaves

Instructions:

1. In a bowl, whisk the eggs with a pinch of salt and pepper.
2. Heat the garlic-infused olive oil in a non-stick frying pan over medium heat.
3. Pour in the eggs and scramble them lightly with a spatula, cooking until just set.
4. Warm the gluten-free tortilla wrap briefly in the oven or on a dry pan.
5. Spread the scrambled eggs down the center of the tortilla wrap.
6. Sprinkle the shredded cheddar cheese over the eggs.
7. Add the spinach leaves on top.
8. Roll up the tortilla wrap, tucking in the ends. Cut in half before serving if desired.

Nutritional Values: Calories: 370 | Protein: 20g | Carbohydrates: 22g | Fiber: 4g | Sugar: 2g | Fat: 23g

Note: If you have a lactose intolerance, ensure you use lactose-free cheese. If you cannot find a suitable gluten-free tortilla, you could use a gluten-free bread alternative.

Preparation Time: 5 minutes | Cooking Time: 15 minutes | Serves: 2

Ingredients:

- 1 cup quinoa
- 2 cups almond milk or another non-dairy milk
- 1 tablespoon pure maple syrup
- 1/2 teaspoon pure vanilla extract
- Pinch of salt
- Optional toppings: a small handful of blueberries, sliced strawberries, and a sprinkle of cinnamon

Instructions:

1. Rinse the quinoa under chilly water until the water runs clear.
2. In a saucepan, combine the quinoa and almond milk. Bring to a boil.
3. Reduce the heat to low, cover the saucepan, and let it simmer for 15 minutes or until the quinoa is tender and has absorbed most of the milk.
4. Stir in the maple syrup, vanilla extract, and a pinch of salt.
5. Divide the quinoa porridge into bowls and add your chosen toppings.

Nutritional Values: Calories: 320 | Protein: 10g | Carbohydrates: 52g | Fiber: 6g | Sugar: 8g | Fat: 8g

Note: Most non-dairy milks are low FODMAP, but brands can vary. If you have a nut allergy, you can substitute oat milk or rice milk for the almond milk. As a sweetener, we use maple syrup, but you can use another low FODMAP sweetener if preferred.

7. BUCKWHEAT BANANA MUFFINS (V)

Preparation Time: 15 minutes | Cooking Time: 25 minutes | Makes: 12 muffins

Ingredients:

- 2 cups buckwheat flour
- 1 teaspoon baking soda
- 1/2 teaspoon salt
- 1/2 cup pure maple syrup
- 1/3 cup olive oil
- 4 ripe bananas, mashed
- 1/4 cup almond milk (or another non-dairy milk)
- 1 teaspoon pure vanilla extract
- Optional toppings: a sprinkle of chia seeds or pumpkin seeds

Instructions:

1. Preheat your oven to 350°F (180°C) and line a muffin tin with paper liners.
2. In a large bowl, combine the buckwheat flour, baking soda, and salt.
3. In a separate bowl, mix the maple syrup, olive oil, mashed bananas, almond milk, and vanilla extract.
4. Gradually add the wet ingredients to the dry ingredients, mixing just until combined.
5. Divide the batter evenly among the muffin cups. If desired, sprinkle the tops with chia seeds or pumpkin seeds.
6. Bake for 25 minutes, or until a toothpick inserted into the center of a muffin comes out clean.
7. Let the muffins cool in the tin for 5 minutes, then transfer them to a wire rack to cool completely.

Nutritional Values: Calories: 220 | Protein: 4g | Carbohydrates: 36g | Fiber: 4g | Sugar: 16g | Fat: 7g

Note: For a nut-free version, substitute the almond milk with another suitable non-dairy milk, such as rice milk or oat milk.

8. FRUIT & NUT GRANOLA WITH LACTOSE-FREE YOGURT (V)

Preparation Time: 10 minutes | Cooking Time: 30 minutes | Makes: 6 servings

Ingredients:

- 2 cups oats (make sure they are certified gluten-free if necessary)
- 1/2 cup walnuts, chopped
- 1/2 cup pecans, chopped
- 1/4 cup pumpkin seeds
- 1/4 cup sunflower seeds
- 2 tablespoons chia seeds
- 2 tablespoons pure maple syrup
- 2 tablespoons olive oil
- 1/2 cup dried cranberries (with no added sugar or other high FODMAP ingredients)
- 1/2 cup dried blueberries (with no added sugar or other high FODMAP ingredients)
- 6 cups lactose-free yogurt for serving

Instructions:

1. Preheat your oven to 300°F (150°C) and line a baking sheet with parchment paper.
2. In a large bowl, combine the oats, walnuts, pecans, pumpkin seeds, sunflower seeds, and chia seeds. Drizzle the maple syrup and olive oil over the top and mix until well coated.
3. Spread the granola mixture out on the prepared baking sheet in an even layer.
4. Bake for 30 minutes, stirring every 10 minutes, until the granola is golden and toasted. Allow the granola to cool completely.
5. Once cooled, mix in the dried cranberries and blueberries.
6. To serve, portion out 1 cup of lactose-free yogurt and top with a generous handful of the granola.

Nutritional Values: Calories: 420 | Protein: 15g | Carbohydrates: 45g | Fiber: 7g | Sugar: 20g | Fat: 21g

Note: You can replace the nuts with seeds for a nut-free version. Check the labels on dried fruits to ensure no high FODMAP ingredients are added.

| | |

9. HEALTHY SPINACH AND TOMATO OMELETTE

Preparation Time: 5 minutes | Cooking Time: 10 minutes | Makes: 1 serving

Ingredients:

- 2 large eggs
- 1/4 cup fresh spinach, chopped
- 1/4 cup common tomatoes (not cherry or Roma), chopped
- 1 tablespoon olive oil
- 1/8 teaspoon salt
- 1/8 teaspoon ground black pepper
- 2 tablespoons lactose-free cheese (optional, or use a suitable non-dairy cheese alternative if intolerant)

Instructions:

1. Crack the eggs into a bowl, add a pinch of salt and pepper, and whisk until well combined.
2. Heat the olive oil over medium heat in a non-stick frying pan.
3. Add the chopped spinach to the pan, and sauté for a couple of minutes until it wilts.
4. Pour the whisked eggs over the spinach, tilt the pan to spread the eggs evenly over the bottom.
5. Sprinkle the chopped tomatoes evenly over the egg.
6. If using, sprinkle the lactose-free cheese or non-dairy cheese alternative over the top.
7. Cover the pan with a lid and cook on a low heat for a few minutes until the eggs are set and the cheese has melted.
8. Fold the omelette in half and serve hot.

Nutritional Values: Calories: 280 | Protein: 16g | Carbohydrates: 4g | Fiber: 1g | Sugar: 2g | Fat: 22g

Note: The specific type of tomato was specified as common tomatoes are low in FODMAPs while cherry and Roma tomatoes are not. Always read labels for any cheese to ensure it is lactose-free or choose a suitable non-dairy cheese alternative if necessary.

10. GLUTEN-FREE WAFFLES WITH MAPLE SYRUP (V)

Preparation Time: 15 minutes | Cooking Time: 15 minutes | Makes: 4 servings

Ingredients:

- 2 cups gluten-free flour blend
- 1 tablespoon sugar
- 1 tablespoon baking powder
- 1/2 teaspoon salt
- 2 large eggs
- 1 3/4 cups lactose-free milk or suitable non-dairy milk (like almond or rice milk)
- 1/2 cup vegetable oil
- 1 teaspoon pure vanilla extract
- 100% pure maple syrup, for serving
- Optional toppings: blueberries, bananas, or strawberries

Instructions:

1. Preheat your waffle iron according to the manufacturer's instructions.
2. In a large bowl, mix together the gluten-free flour, sugar, baking powder, and salt.
3. In another bowl, whisk together the eggs, lactose-free milk, vegetable oil, and vanilla extract.
4. Pour the wet ingredients into the dry ingredients and stir until just combined.
5. Ladle the batter into the preheated waffle iron and cook according to the manufacturer's instructions until golden brown.
6. Serve the waffles hot, drizzled with pure maple syrup and optional toppings of blueberries, bananas, or strawberries.

Nutritional Values: Calories: 460 | Protein: 9g | Carbohydrates: 57g | Fiber: 3g | Sugar: 10g | Fat: 23g

Note: Be sure to read labels to ensure that the gluten-free flour blend and non-dairy milk are indeed gluten and lactose-free. Choose for a milk substitute like almond milk or rice milk if lactose intolerant. Always choose 100% pure maple syrup, as some brands may add high-FODMAP sweeteners. Fruits like blueberries, bananas, and strawberries are low in FODMAPs and can be used as toppings.

11. Stuffed Bell Peppers with Scrambled Eggs

Preparation Time: 10 minutes | Cooking Time: 15 minutes | Makes: 4 servings

Ingredients:

- 4 large bell peppers (any color)
- 8 large eggs
- 1/4 cup lactose-free milk or suitable non-dairy milk (like almond or rice milk)
- Salt and pepper to taste
- 2 tablespoons olive oil
- Optional garnish: fresh chopped parsley or chives

Instructions:

1. Cut the tops off the bell peppers and remove the seeds. Set aside.
2. In a bowl, whisk together the eggs, lactose-free milk, salt, and pepper.
3. Heat the olive oil in a large non-stick skillet over medium heat. Add the egg mixture and cook, stirring often, until scrambled and just set. Remove from heat.
4. Using a spoon, divide the scrambled eggs evenly among the hollowed bell peppers.
5. If desired, garnish with fresh chopped parsley or chives before serving.

Nutritional Values: Calories: 230 | Protein: 13g | Carbohydrates: 9g | Fiber: 3g | Sugar: 6g | Fat: 16g

Note: This recipe is a wonderful way to enjoy a protein-packed breakfast without triggering IBS symptoms. Always check labels to make sure that your non-dairy milk does not contain high FODMAP additives. If you are sensitive to eggs, you can try using a suitable egg substitute. However, be aware that egg substitutes can sometimes contain high FODMAP ingredients, so it is essential to read labels. Always choose fresh herbs for garnishing, as dried herbs can sometimes contain high FODMAP ingredients.

12. Buckwheat and Blueberry Breakfast Bowl (VG)

Preparation Time: 10 minutes | Cooking Time: 15 minutes | Makes: 2 servings

Ingredients:

- 1 cup of buckwheat groats
- 2 cups of water
- 1 cup of fresh blueberries
- 1 tablespoon of chia seeds
- 2 tablespoons of pure maple syrup
- 1 cup of unsweetened almond milk
- Optional toppings: A small number of sliced almonds or pumpkin seeds

Instructions:

1. Rinse the buckwheat groats thoroughly under freezing water.
2. In a pot, combine the buckwheat groats and water. Bring to a boil, then reduce the heat to low and let it simmer for about 15 minutes until the buckwheat is tender and the water is absorbed. Remove from heat.
3. Divide the cooked buckwheat between two bowls.
4. Top each bowl with half of the blueberries and half of the chia seeds. Drizzle each serving with 1 tablespoon of maple syrup.
5. Pour 1/2 cup of unsweetened almond milk over each bowl.
6. If desired, add a sprinkling of sliced almonds or pumpkin seeds for extra crunch.
7. Serve immediately and enjoy your nourishing and delicious low FODMAP breakfast.

Nutritional Values: Calories: 370 | Protein: 9g | Carbohydrates: 70g | Fiber: 9g | Sugar: 20g | Fat: 7g

Note: This recipe is vegan, gluten-free, and low in FODMAPs. Buckwheat, despite its name, is a gluten-free grain. Blueberries are low FODMAP in servings of a heaped tablespoon (28g) per sitting. A larger serving may contain higher levels of fructans. Be mindful of your own tolerance level.

Preparation Time: 5 minutes | Cooking Time: 0 minutes | Makes: 1 serving

Ingredients:

- 1 medium ripe banana (around 100g is low FODMAP)
- 2 tablespoons of peanut butter (without additives)
- 1 cup of unsweetened almond milk
- 1 tablespoon of chia seeds
- 1 tablespoon of pure maple syrup (optional)
- A handful of ice cubes

Instructions:

1. Peel the banana and slice it into chunks.
2. Add the banana chunks, peanut butter, unsweetened almond milk, chia seeds, and maple syrup (if using) into a blender.
3. Blend until the mixture is smooth and creamy.
4. Add the ice cubes and blend again until the smoothie is chilled.
5. Pour the smoothie into a glass and serve immediately.
6. Enjoy this delicious, satisfying, and low FODMAP vegan smoothie!

Nutritional Values: Calories: 390 | Protein: 12g | Carbohydrates: 37g | Fiber: 9g | Sugar: 18g | Fat: 23g

Note: This recipe is vegan, gluten-free, and low FODMAP. Peanut butter is low FODMAP in servings of 2 tablespoons per sitting. Larger servings can contain higher levels of both fructans and GOS. Be mindful of your own tolerance level.

Preparation Time: 10 minutes | Cooking Time: 10 minutes | Makes: 1 serving

Ingredients:

- 1 large egg
- 1 low-FODMAP tortilla (such as a corn tortilla)
- 1/4 cup diced bell peppers
- 1/4 cup diced tomatoes
- 1/4 cup shredded Cheddar cheese (lactose-free if necessary)
- 1 tablespoon of olive oil
- Salt and pepper to taste

Instructions:

1. In a non-stick pan, heat the olive oil over medium heat.
2. Add the bell peppers and tomatoes to the pan and sauté until they are soft.
3. Crack the egg into a bowl and whisk it lightly with a fork. Pour the whisked egg into the pan with the vegetables.
4. Stir the mixture until the egg is cooked to your liking. Season with salt and pepper.
5. Warm the tortilla in a separate pan over medium heat or in a microwave for about 15 seconds.
6. Place the cooked egg and vegetable mixture onto the center of the tortilla.
7. Sprinkle the shredded Cheddar cheese on top.
8. Fold the bottom of the tortilla over the filling, then fold in the sides and roll it up tightly.
9. Serve your FODMAP-friendly breakfast burrito warm and enjoy!

Nutritional Values: Calories: 410 | Protein: 17g | Carbohydrates: 25g | Fiber: 4g | Sugar: 4g | Fat: 27g

Note: This recipe is gluten-free and low FODMAP. If you have lactose intolerance, ensure the cheddar cheese you use is lactose-free. The hard, aged cheeses like cheddar are naturally low in lactose. Always check the ingredients for added high FODMAP items.

15. Oatmeal with Cinnamon and Grated Apple (VG)

Preparation Time: 5 minutes | Cooking Time: 10 minutes | Makes: 1 serving

Ingredients:

- 1/2 cup gluten-free oats
- 1 cup almond milk (ensure it is a low-FODMAP variety)
- 1 small unripe banana, sliced
- 1/4 teaspoon cinnamon
- 1/2 medium green apple, grated

Instructions:

1. In a small pot, combine the oats, almond milk, and sliced banana.
2. Bring the mixture to a boil over medium-high heat, then reduce to a simmer.
3. Cook, stirring often, for about 10 minutes or until the oats have absorbed most of the liquid and are creamy.
4. Stir in the cinnamon.
5. Transfer the cooked oatmeal to a bowl and top with the grated green apple.
6. Serve warm and enjoy!

Nutritional Values: Calories: 280 | Protein: 6g | Carbohydrates: 55g | Fiber: 8g | Sugar: 18g | Fat: 5g

Note: This recipe is vegan, gluten-free, and low FODMAP. Please ensure the almond milk you use is a low-FODMAP variety, as some types of almond milk can contain high-FODMAP additives like inulin. For those with apple intolerance, the green apple can be replaced with a low-FODMAP fruit like strawberries or blueberries. Always check the ingredients for added high FODMAP items.

16. Strawberry and Chia Seed Jam on Gluten-Free Toast (V)

Preparation Time: 10 minutes | Cooking Time: 15 minutes | Makes: 6 servings

Ingredients:

- 2 cups fresh strawberries, hulled and quartered
- 2 tablespoons pure maple syrup
- 2 tablespoons chia seeds
- 1 teaspoon vanilla extract
- 6 slices of gluten-free bread

Instructions:

1. In a medium-sized saucepan, add the strawberries and maple syrup. Cook over medium heat until the strawberries start to break down, about 10 minutes.
2. Using a potato masher or a fork, gently crush the strawberries to your desired consistency.
3. Stir in the chia seeds and continue to cook the mixture for another 5 minutes, or until it thickens.
4. Remove from heat and stir in the vanilla extract. Let the jam cool for a few minutes.
5. While the jam is cooling, toast the gluten-free bread slices until golden brown.
6. Spread a generous amount of strawberry chia seed jam on each slice of toast. Serve immediately and enjoy!

Nutritional Values: Calories: 130 | Protein: 3g | Carbohydrates: 22g | Fiber: 4g | Sugar: 10g | Fat: 3g

Note: This recipe is vegan and low FODMAP. As always, ensure the gluten-free bread you use is a low-FODMAP variety, as some types can contain high-FODMAP ingredients. For those with strawberry intolerance, the strawberries can be replaced with blueberries, which are a low-FODMAP fruit. Always check the ingredients for added high FODMAP items.

17. Bacon and Egg Breakfast Muffins

Preparation Time: 10 minutes | Cooking Time: 20 minutes | Makes: 6 servings

Ingredients:

- 6 large eggs
- 6 strips of bacon, cooked and crumbled
- 1/2 cup diced green bell peppers
- 1/2 cup diced tomatoes
- 1/4 cup chopped fresh chives
- Salt and pepper to taste
- 1/2 cup shredded cheddar cheese (use a lactose-free variety if lactose intolerant)

Instructions:

1. Preheat your oven to 375°F (190°C). Grease a muffin tin or line it with silicone muffin cups.
2. In a medium bowl, whisk the eggs. Add the crumbled bacon, diced bell peppers, diced tomatoes, chives, and salt and pepper. Mix until everything is well combined.
3. Divide the egg mixture evenly among the muffin cups.
4. Sprinkle the shredded cheddar cheese on top of each muffin cup.
5. Bake for 20 minutes, or until the muffins are set in the middle.
6. Let them cool for a few minutes before removing from the muffin tin. Serve warm and enjoy!

Nutritional Values: Calories: 170 | Protein: 12g | Carbohydrates: 3g | Fiber: 0.5g | Sugar: 2g | Fat: 12g

Note: This recipe is low FODMAP. If you are lactose intolerant, make sure to use a lactose-free cheddar cheese. If you are sensitive to the green bell peppers, you can replace them with a similar low FODMAP vegetable, like spinach. As always, ensure the bacon is free from high FODMAP ingredients like garlic and onion.

18. Almond Milk Overnight Oats with Raspberries (VG)

Preparation Time: 10 minutes | Soaking Time: Overnight | Makes: 2 servings

Ingredients:

- 1 cup gluten-free rolled oats
- 2 cups unsweetened almond milk
- 2 tablespoons chia seeds
- 2 tablespoons pure maple syrup
- 1/2 cup fresh blueberries
- A handful of chopped almonds (small quantity, within the FODMAP limit)

Instructions:

1. In a large bowl, mix the rolled oats, almond milk, chia seeds, and maple syrup.
2. Divide the mixture evenly between two mason jars or containers with lids.
3. Seal the jars and refrigerate overnight, or for at least 6 hours.
4. In the morning, give the oats a good stir. The chia seeds will have absorbed some of the almond milk, making the mixture thick.
5. Top each serving with a handful of fresh blueberries and chopped almonds. Enjoy cold or heat in the microwave for 1-2 minutes if you prefer it warm.

Nutritional Values: Calories: 350 | Protein: 10g | Carbohydrates: 50g | Fiber: 10g | Sugar: 15g | Fat: 12g

Note: This recipe contains a small number of almonds which can be high in FODMAPs if consumed in copious amounts. If you have a sensitivity to almonds, you could omit them or replace with a sprinkling of pumpkin seeds. Also, please note that raspberries are replaced with blueberries as the former are high in FODMAPs. As always, ensure all your ingredients are low FODMAP, including your almond milk (should be free of high FODMAP additives like inulin or chicory root fiber).

19. Sautéed Tomatoes and Spinach on Sourdough Toast (V)

Preparation Time: 10 minutes | Cooking Time: 10 minutes | Makes: 1 serving

Ingredients:

- 2 slices gluten-free sourdough bread
- 1 tablespoon olive oil
- 1 cup cherry tomatoes
- 1 cup baby spinach leaves
- Salt to taste
- Black pepper to taste

Instructions:

1. Toast the gluten-free sourdough bread in a toaster until golden brown.
2. In a non-stick frying pan, heat the olive oil over medium heat.
3. Add the cherry tomatoes to the pan and sauté for about 5 minutes, or until they start to burst and soften.
4. Add the spinach to the pan and continue to sauté until the spinach wilts, this should take about 1-2 minutes.
5. Season with salt and black pepper to taste.
6. Spoon the sautéed tomatoes and spinach over the toasted gluten-free sourdough slices and serve immediately.

Nutritional Values: Calories: 330 | Protein: 8g | Carbohydrates: 40g | Fiber: 6g | Sugar: 6g | Fat: 16g

Note: Ensure your gluten-free sourdough bread is suitable for a low FODMAP diet. If you are sensitive to cherry tomatoes, you can replace them with a suitable low FODMAP vegetable like bell peppers or zucchini.

20. Quinoa and Zucchini Fritters (VG)

Preparation Time: 15 minutes | Cooking Time: 15 minutes | Makes: 4 servings

Ingredients:

- 1 cup quinoa
- 2 cups water
- 2 medium zucchinis, grated
- 1/4 cup chives, finely chopped
- 1/4 cup dill, finely chopped
- 1/2 cup gluten-free all-purpose flour
- Salt to taste
- Pepper to taste
- 3 tablespoons olive oil

Instructions:

1. Rinse the quinoa under cold water until the water runs clear.
2. In a saucepan, bring the water to a boil. Add the quinoa, reduce the heat to low, cover, and simmer for 15 minutes, or until all the water is absorbed. Remove from heat and let it cool.
3. In a large bowl, combine the cooked quinoa, grated zucchini, chives, dill, and gluten-free flour. Season with salt and pepper to taste.
4. Stir until everything is well combined.
5. Shape the mixture into small patties.
6. Heat the olive oil in a non-stick frying pan over medium heat.
7. Cook the fritters in batches for 3-4 minutes on each side, or until golden brown.
8. Transfer the fritters to a plate lined with paper towels to drain excess oil.
9. Serve warm with a side salad if desired.

Nutritional Values: Calories: 290 | Protein: 8g | Carbohydrates: 38g | Fiber: 6g | Sugar: 3g | Fat: 11g

Note: Make sure your gluten-free flour does not contain high FODMAP ingredients like inulin, apple or pear juice, or honey.

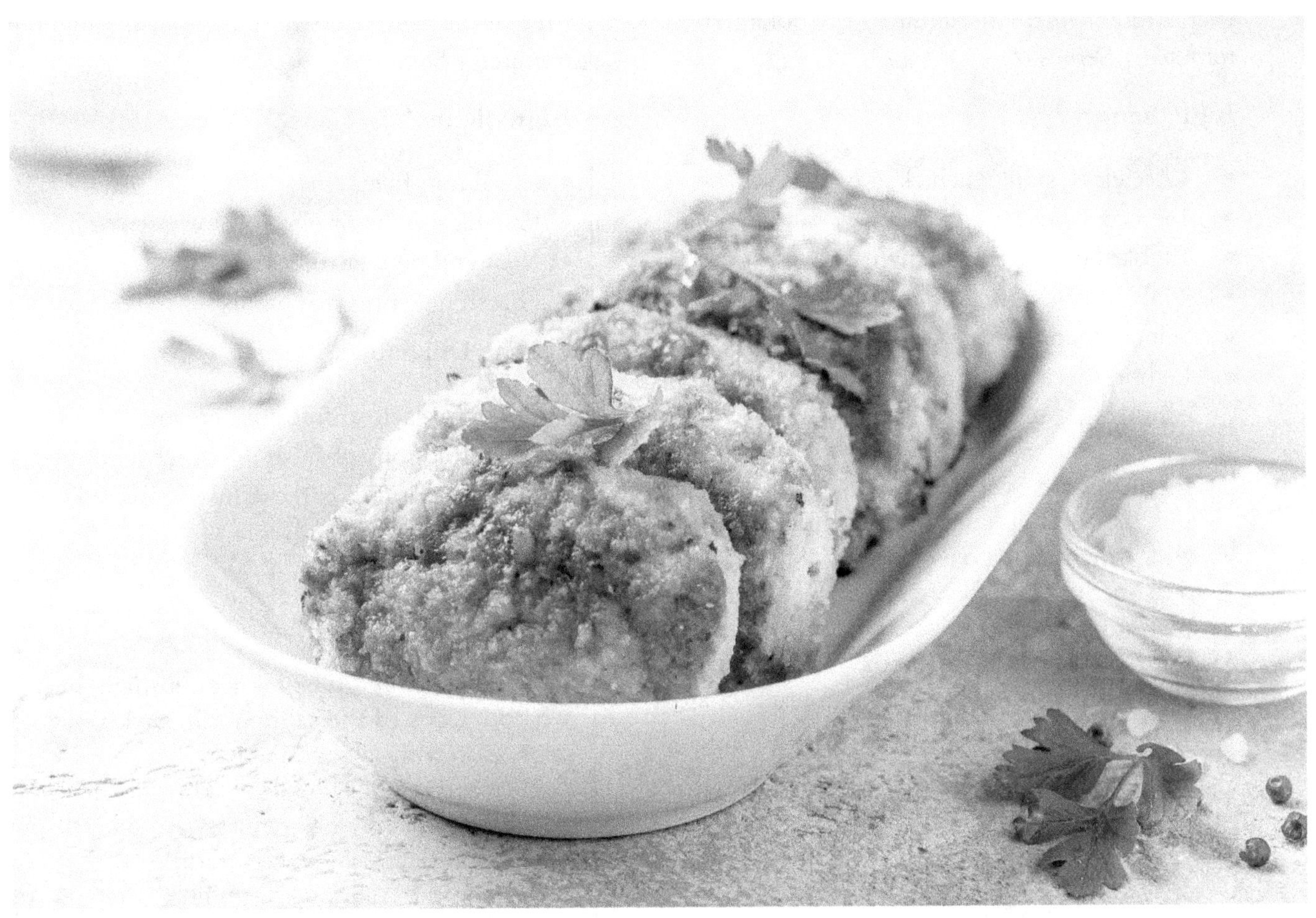

Preparation time: 10 minutes | Cooking time: 25 minutes | Serves: 4

Ingredients:

- 4 boneless, skinless chicken breasts
- 1 lemon (for zest and juice)
- 2 tablespoons of fresh thyme leaves
- 2 tablespoons of garlic-infused olive oil
- Salt and pepper to taste
- Lemon slices and extra thyme sprigs for garnish

Instructions:

1. Preheat your oven to 200°C (392°F). In a bowl, mix the zest and juice of the lemon, thyme leaves, and garlic-infused olive oil.
2. Season the chicken breasts with salt and pepper on both sides, then place them in a baking dish.
3. Pour the lemon-thyme-oil mixture over the chicken breasts, ensuring they are fully coated.
4. Bake the chicken in the preheated oven for about 20-25 minutes, or until the chicken is fully cooked through and no longer pink in the middle.
5. Once done, remove from the oven and let rest for a few minutes.
6. Serve the chicken hot, garnished with lemon slices and extra thyme sprigs if desired.

Nutritional Values: Calories: 250 | Carbohydrates: 3g | Protein: 30g | Fat: 12g | Fiber: 1g | Sugar: 1g

Preparation time: 10 minutes | Cooking time: 15 minutes | Serves: 4

Ingredients:

- 4 salmon fillets
- 2 tablespoons of olive oil
- Salt and pepper to taste
- Fresh dill sprigs for garnish

For the Dill Sauce:

- 1 cup of lactose-free sour cream
- 2 tablespoons of fresh dill, finely chopped
- 1 tablespoon of garlic-infused olive oil
- Juice of half a lemon
- Salt and pepper to taste

Instructions:

1. Preheat your grill on medium-high heat. Brush both sides of the salmon fillets with olive oil and season with salt and pepper.
2. Place the salmon fillets skin-side down on the grill. Cook for 6-8 minutes per side, or until the salmon flakes easily with a fork.
3. While the salmon is grilling, prepare the dill sauce. In a bowl, combine the lactose-free sour cream, fresh dill, garlic-infused olive oil, lemon juice, salt, and pepper. Stir until well combined.
4. Once the salmon is cooked, remove from the grill, and let it rest for a few minutes.
5. Serve the grilled salmon with a generous dollop of dill sauce on top. Garnish with fresh dill sprigs if desired.

Nutritional Values: Calories: 370 | Carbohydrates: 3g | Protein: 34g | Fat: 24g | Fiber: 1g | Sugar: 1g

Preparation time: 15 minutes | Cooking time: 15 minutes | Serves: 4

Ingredients:

- 500g skinless chicken breast, cut into thin strips
- 1 tablespoon garlic-infused olive oil
- 1 medium-size bell pepper, thinly sliced
- 1 medium-size zucchini, thinly sliced
- 2 medium-size carrots, thinly sliced
- 2 tablespoons low-sodium soy sauce (gluten-free)
- 1 tablespoon rice vinegar
- 1 tablespoon fresh ginger, grated
- 1 tablespoon sesame seeds
- 1 tablespoon chives, finely chopped

Instructions:

1. Heat the garlic-infused olive oil in a large wok or skillet over medium-high heat. Add the chicken strips and cook until lightly browned and no longer pink in the center. Remove the chicken and set aside.
2. In the same wok, add the bell pepper, zucchini, and carrots. Stir-fry for about 3-4 minutes, until the vegetables are slightly tender but still crispy.
3. In a small bowl, combine the low-sodium soy sauce, rice vinegar, and fresh ginger. Stir well to combine.
4. Return the cooked chicken to the wok. Pour over the soy sauce mixture and stir well to combine. Cook for another 2-3 minutes, until everything is well coated and heated through.
5. Sprinkle the stir-fry with sesame seeds and finely chopped chives just before serving.

Nutritional Values: Calories: 260 | Carbohydrates: 10g | Protein: 30g | Fat: 10g | Fiber: 3g | Sugar: 6g

Preparation time: 10 minutes | Cooking time: 20 minutes | Serves: 4

Ingredients:

- 1 cup quinoa
- 2 cups low FODMAP vegetable broth
- 1 medium zucchini, sliced lengthwise
- 1 medium bell pepper, sliced
- 2 medium carrots, sliced
- 1 tablespoon garlic-infused olive oil
- 2 tablespoons fresh lemon juice
- 1 tablespoon fresh chopped basil
- Salt and pepper to taste

Instructions:

1. Rinse quinoa under icy water until the water runs clear. Combine quinoa and vegetable broth in a medium saucepan. Bring to a boil, then reduce heat to low, cover, and simmer for 15 minutes, or until all liquid is absorbed.
2. While quinoa is cooking, heat a grill or grill pan over medium-high heat. Toss zucchini, bell pepper, and carrots with the garlic-infused olive oil. Grill vegetables for about 3-4 minutes per side, until slightly charred and tender.
3. In a large bowl, combine the cooked quinoa, grilled vegetables, lemon juice, and fresh basil. Season with salt and pepper to taste. Toss to combine well.
4. Serve warm or chilled, as preferred.

Nutritional Values: Calories: 220 | Carbohydrates: 35g | Protein: 8g | Fat: 6g | Fiber: 6g | Sugar: 4g

25. TUNA AND RICE SALAD WITH LEMON VINAIGRETTE

Preparation time: 10 minutes | Cooking time: 20 minutes | Serves: 4

Ingredients:

- 1 cup basmati rice
- 2 cups low FODMAP vegetable broth
- 1 can (5 oz) tuna in water, drained
- 1 cup cherry tomatoes, halved
- 1/2 cup sliced cucumber
- 2 green onions (green parts only), finely chopped
- 1/4 cup chopped fresh parsley

For the Lemon Vinaigrette:

- 3 tablespoons extra-virgin olive oil
- 2 tablespoons fresh lemon juice
- 1 tablespoon Dijon mustard
- Salt and pepper to taste

Instructions:

1. Rinse the basmati rice under cold water until the water runs clear. Combine the rice and vegetable broth in a medium saucepan. Bring to a boil, then reduce the heat to low, cover, and simmer for about 15-20 minutes, or until all the liquid is absorbed.
2. In a large bowl, combine the cooked rice, tuna, cherry tomatoes, cucumber, green onions, and parsley.
3. For the vinaigrette, whisk together the olive oil, lemon juice, and Dijon mustard in a small bowl. Season with salt and pepper to taste.
4. Pour the vinaigrette over the rice and tuna mixture and toss to combine well. Serve at room temperature or chilled, as preferred.

Nutritional Values: Calories: 280 | Carbohydrates: 40g | Protein: 14g | Fat: 7g | Fiber: 2g | Sugar: 2g

26. GLUTEN-FREE PASTA WITH GARLIC INFUSED OLIVE OIL AND CHILI (V)

Preparation time: 5 minutes | Cooking time: 15 minutes | Serves: 4

Ingredients:

- 8 oz gluten-free pasta
- 1/4 cup garlic-infused olive oil
- 1/2 teaspoon red chili flakes
- Salt and pepper to taste
- Fresh basil leaves for garnish
- Lemon zest for garnish

Instructions:

1. Cook the gluten-free pasta in a large pot of boiling salted water according to the package instructions until al dente. Drain and set aside.
2. Meanwhile, heat the garlic-infused olive oil in a large pan over medium heat. Add the red chili flakes and cook for 1-2 minutes, being careful not to burn them.
3. Add the cooked pasta to the pan and toss to coat in the olive oil. Season with salt and pepper to taste.
4. Serve the pasta in individual bowls, garnished with fresh basil leaves and lemon zest.

Nutritional Values: Calories: 370 | Carbohydrates: 53g | Protein: 7g | Fat: 15g | Fiber: 3g | Sugar: 2g

Preparation time: 15 minutes | Cooking time: 20 minutes | Serves: 4

Ingredients:

- 1 lb lean ground beef
- 1 tablespoon olive oil
- 1 tablespoon cumin
- 1 teaspoon smoked paprika
- 1 teaspoon dried oregano
- Salt and pepper to taste
- 8 corn tortillas
- 1 cup chopped tomatoes
- 1 cup shredded lettuce
- 1/2 cup diced cucumbers
- 1/2 cup diced red bell peppers
- 1/2 cup lactose-free cheddar cheese, shredded

Instructions:

1. Heat the olive oil in a large pan over medium heat. Add the ground beef and cook until browned, about 5-7 minutes. Drain the excess fat.
2. Add the cumin, smoked paprika, dried oregano, salt, and pepper to the beef and stir well. Cook for another 2-3 minutes.
3. Warm the corn tortillas in a dry pan over medium heat until they are pliable.
4. To assemble the tacos, divide the ground beef evenly among the tortillas. Top with the chopped tomatoes, shredded lettuce, diced cucumbers, and diced red bell peppers. Sprinkle with lactose-free cheddar cheese.
5. Serve immediately.

Nutritional Values: Calories: 450 | Carbohydrates: 33g | Protein: 28g | Fat: 23g | Fiber: 5g | Sugar: 3g

Preparation time: 15 minutes | Cooking time: 10 minutes | Serves: 4

Ingredients:

- 4 medium zucchinis
- 1 pound shrimp, peeled and deveined
- 1 tablespoon olive oil
- Salt and pepper to taste
- 1 teaspoon dried basil
- 1 tablespoon fresh lemon juice
- 1/4 cup FODMAP-safe chicken broth
- 1/2 cup cherry tomatoes, halved
- 2 tablespoons chopped fresh parsley

Instructions:

1. Use a spiralizer to cut the zucchini into noodle shapes. Set aside.
2. Heat the olive oil in a large pan over medium heat. Add the shrimp and cook until pink, about 2-3 minutes per side. Remove the shrimp from the pan and set aside.
3. In the same pan, add the zucchini noodles and cook for 2-3 minutes, or until just tender. Remove from the pan and set aside with the shrimp.
4. In the pan, add the dried basil, lemon juice, and chicken broth. Bring to a simmer and cook for 2 minutes.
5. Return the shrimp and zucchini noodles to the pan, add the cherry tomatoes, and toss everything together to combine.
6. Season with salt and pepper to taste, and garnish with the chopped fresh parsley.
7. Serve immediately.

Nutritional Values: Calories: 170 | Carbohydrates: 10g | Protein: 20g | Fat: 5g | Fiber: 2g | Sugar: 7g

Preparation time: 20 minutes | Cooking time: 15 minutes | Serves: 4

Ingredients:

- 4 boneless, skinless chicken breasts
- 1 tablespoon olive oil
- Salt and pepper to taste
- 2 medium cucumbers, diced
- 1 red bell pepper, diced
- 20 cherry tomatoes, halved
- 1/2 cup pitted kalamata olives
- 4 ounces feta cheese, cubed (Lactose-free for intolerant individuals)
- 2 tablespoons fresh lemon juice
- 1/4 cup extra virgin olive oil
- 1 tablespoon dried oregano
- 2 tablespoons chopped fresh parsley

Instructions:

1. Preheat a grill or grill pan over medium-high heat. Brush the chicken breasts with the olive oil and season with salt and pepper. Grill for 6-7 minutes on each side, or until cooked through. Let rest for a few minutes, then slice.
2. In a large bowl, combine the cucumbers, bell pepper, cherry tomatoes, olives, and feta cheese.
3. In a small bowl, whisk together the lemon juice, olive oil, oregano, and parsley. Season with salt and pepper to taste.
4. Pour the dressing over the salad and toss to combine. Top with the sliced grilled chicken.
5. Serve immediately or refrigerate until ready to eat.

Nutritional Values: Calories: 400 | Carbohydrates: 10g | Protein: 32g | Fat: 27g | Fiber: 3g | Sugar: 5g

Preparation time: 15 minutes | Cooking time: 10 minutes | Serves: 4

Ingredients:

- 8 large eggs
- 1/4 cup mayonnaise (Lactose-free for intolerant individuals)
- 1 tablespoon Dijon mustard
- Salt and pepper to taste
- 2 tablespoons fresh dill, chopped
- 1 small cucumber, diced
- 1 medium carrot, grated
- 8 large lettuce leaves (romaine or butter lettuce)

Instructions:

1. Place the eggs in a saucepan and cover with chilly water. Bring to a boil, then cover, remove from heat, and let stand for 9 minutes. After 9 minutes, drain and cool the eggs in ice water. Once cool, peel and chop the eggs.
2. In a bowl, combine the mayonnaise, Dijon mustard, salt, pepper, and dill. Add the chopped eggs, cucumber, and grated carrot to the bowl, gently mixing until everything is well coated with the dressing.
3. Lay out the lettuce leaves and evenly distribute the egg salad among the leaves.
4. Roll the lettuce leaves around the filling, tuck in the ends and serve.

Nutritional Values: Calories: 250 | Carbohydrates: 5g | Protein: 13g | Fat: 20g | Fiber: 1g | Sugar: 3g

Preparation time: 10 minutes | Cooking time: 15 minutes | Serves: 4

Ingredients:

- 4 cod fillets (about 6 oz each)
- 2 tablespoons olive oil
- Salt and pepper to taste
- 2 lemons, zest, and juice
- 4 cloves of garlic, finely chopped (use a garlic-infused oil for a low FODMAP option)
- 4 tablespoons fresh parsley, finely chopped

Instructions:

1. Preheat your oven to 400°F (200°C). Line a baking sheet with parchment paper.
2. Rub the cod fillets with 1 tablespoon of olive oil and season with salt and pepper. Place the fillets on the prepared baking sheet.
3. In a small bowl, mix the remaining olive oil, lemon zest, lemon juice, and chopped garlic (or garlic-infused oil).
4. Drizzle the lemon mixture over the cod fillets. Bake for about 12-15 minutes, or until the fish flakes easily with a fork.
5. Garnish with fresh parsley before serving. Enjoy with a side of steamed vegetables or a simple green salad for a complete low FODMAP meal.

Nutritional Values: Calories: 190 | Carbohydrates: 2g | Protein: 30g | Fat: 7g | Fiber: 1g | Sugar: 1g

Preparation time: 10 minutes | Cooking time: 20 minutes | Serves: 4

Ingredients:

- 4 steak cuts of your choice (about 6 oz each)
- Salt and pepper to taste
- 1 tablespoon garlic-infused oil
- 2 tablespoons olive oil, divided
- 1 lb fresh green beans, trimmed
- 1 teaspoon red pepper flakes (optional)

Instructions:

1. Preheat your grill to medium-high heat.
2. Season the steak cuts with salt and pepper to taste. Drizzle one tablespoon of olive oil over the steaks.
3. Place the steaks on the preheated grill and cook to your preferred level of doneness, about 4-5 minutes per side for medium-rare. Remove from the grill and let rest for a few minutes.
4. Meanwhile, in a large skillet, heat the remaining olive oil and the garlic-infused oil over medium heat. Add the green beans and sauté until they are tender and slightly charred, about 10-12 minutes.
5. If using, sprinkle the red pepper flakes over the green beans and stir to combine.
6. Serve the grilled steaks with a side of the sautéed green beans.

Nutritional Values: Calories: 375 | Carbohydrates: 8g | Protein: 35g | Fat: 23g | Fiber: 3g | Sugar: 4g

Preparation time: 10 minutes | Cooking time: 20 minutes | Serves: 4

Ingredients:

- 2 cups cooked basmati rice (cooled)
- 1 lb raw shrimp, peeled and deveined
- 2 tablespoons garlic-infused oil
- 1 cup diced bell peppers (green and red)
- 1/2 cup diced carrots
- 2 large eggs, beaten
- 2 tablespoons gluten-free soy sauce or tamari
- 2 green onions, sliced (green part only)
- Salt to taste

Instructions:

1. Heat a tablespoon of the garlic-infused oil in a large skillet or wok over medium-high heat. Add the shrimp and cook until pink, about 2-3 minutes. Remove the shrimp from the skillet and set aside.
2. In the same skillet, add the remaining garlic-infused oil. Add the bell peppers and carrots. Cook, stirring occasionally, until the vegetables are tender, about 3-4 minutes.
3. Push the vegetables to one side of the skillet, then add the beaten eggs to the other side. Stir gently until the eggs are fully cooked.
4. Add the cooked rice to the skillet and stir to combine with the vegetables and eggs. Then, stir in the cooked shrimp.
5. Pour the soy sauce or tamari over the rice mixture and stir to combine. Cook for another 2 minutes, until everything is well combined and heated through.
6. Season with salt to taste, garnish with the sliced green onions, and serve.

Nutritional Values: Calories: 370 | Carbohydrates: 42g | Protein: 27g | Fat: 8g | Fiber: 2g | Sugar: 3g

Preparation time: 15 minutes | Cooking time: 30 minutes | Serves: 4

Ingredients:

- 4 boneless, skinless chicken breasts
- 1/4 cup gluten-free tamari or low-sodium soy sauce
- 2 tablespoons maple syrup
- 1 tablespoon rice vinegar
- 1 tablespoon freshly grated ginger
- 1 tablespoon cornstarch
- 1 cup jasmine rice
- 2 cups low-FODMAP vegetable broth or water
- 1 tablespoon garlic-infused oil
- 1 cup diced bell peppers (green and red)
- 1/2 cup diced carrots
- Salt to taste

Instructions:

1. In a bowl, combine tamari or soy sauce, maple syrup, rice vinegar, and ginger. Stir until well combined.
2. Place the chicken breasts in a large zip-top bag and pour the marinade over the chicken. Seal the bag and let the chicken marinate in the fridge for at least 30 minutes, or up to 24 hours.
3. After marinating, remove the chicken from the bag, reserving the marinade. Heat the garlic-infused oil in a skillet over medium-high heat, add the chicken breasts, and cook until browned on both sides and cooked through, about 6-8 minutes per side. Remove the chicken from the skillet and set aside.
4. In the same skillet, add the bell peppers and carrots. Cook until tender, about 5 minutes. Remove from the skillet and set aside.
5. Pour the reserved marinade into the skillet and bring to a simmer. In a small bowl, mix the cornstarch with 2 tablespoons of water to make a slurry, then stir this into the simmering marinade. Continue cooking until the sauce thickens, about 2 minutes.
6. While the vegetables and chicken are cooking, prepare the jasmine rice according to the package instructions, substituting the vegetable broth or water for cooking liquid.

7. To serve, spoon a portion of rice onto each plate, top with a chicken breast and the sautéed vegetables, and drizzle with the thickened teriyaki sauce.

Nutritional Values: Calories: 420 | Carbohydrates: 56g | Protein: 33g | Fat: 7g | Fiber: 3g | Sugar: 10g

35. Quinoa and Tofu Stuffed Peppers (VG)

Preparation time: 15 minutes | Cooking time: 35 minutes | Serves: 4

Ingredients:

- 4 large bell peppers (any color)
- 1 cup quinoa
- 2 cups low-sodium vegetable broth
- 1 block (14 oz.) firm tofu, drained and crumbled
- 1 tablespoon olive oil
- 1/2 cup diced zucchini
- 1/2 cup diced eggplant
- 1 tablespoon garlic-infused oil
- 1 tablespoon fresh chopped basil
- 1 tablespoon fresh chopped parsley
- Salt and pepper to taste

Instructions:

1. Preheat the oven to 375°F (190°C).
2. Cut the tops off the bell peppers and remove the seeds. Place the peppers in a baking dish and set aside.
3. In a saucepan, combine the quinoa and vegetable broth. Bring to a boil, then reduce heat to low, cover, and let simmer for 15 minutes, or until all the broth is absorbed and quinoa is fluffy.
4. While the quinoa is cooking, heat the olive oil in a skillet over medium heat. Add the crumbled tofu, zucchini, and eggplant. Cook until the vegetables are tender and the tofu is slightly golden, about 7-10 minutes.
5. Stir in the cooked quinoa, garlic-infused oil, basil, parsley, and season with salt and pepper.
6. Fill each pepper with the quinoa-tofu mixture. Cover the baking dish with aluminum foil.
7. Bake for 25 minutes. Then, remove the foil and bake for another 10 minutes, or until the peppers are tender and the filling is heated through.
8. Serve hot.

Nutritional Values: Calories: 350 | Carbohydrates: 42g | Protein: 20g | Fat: 13g | Fiber: 7g | Sugar: 7g

36. Grilled Tuna Steaks with Olive Tapenade

Preparation time: 10 minutes | Cooking time: 10 minutes | Serves: 4

Ingredients:

- 4 tuna steaks (about 6 ounces each)
- 1 tablespoon olive oil
- Salt and pepper to taste
- 1 cup mixed pitted olives (such as Kalamata and green olives)
- 1 tablespoon capers
- 1 tablespoon lemon juice
- 2 tablespoons fresh chopped parsley
- 1/4 cup olive oil
- 2 tablespoons chopped fresh basil

Instructions:

1. Preheat the grill to high heat.
2. Brush the tuna steaks with the tablespoon of olive oil and season with salt and pepper.
3. Place the tuna steaks on the grill and cook for about 3-4 minutes on each side or until desired doneness.
4. While the tuna is cooking, make the olive tapenade. In a food processor, combine the olives, capers, lemon juice, parsley, 1/4 cup olive oil, and basil. Pulse until finely chopped but still a little chunky.
5. Once the tuna steaks are done, remove from the grill and let rest for a few minutes.
6. Top each steak with a spoonful of the olive tapenade before serving.

Nutritional Values: Calories: 400 | Carbohydrates: 5g | Protein: 40g | Fat: 25g | Fiber: 1g | Sugar: 0g

Preparation time: 10 minutes | Cooking time: 0 minutes | Serves: 4

Ingredients:

- 8 large lettuce leaves (such as romaine or iceberg)
- 1 pound sliced turkey breast
- 8 slices Swiss cheese
- 1 cucumber, thinly sliced
- 2 medium carrots, peeled and julienned
- 1 red bell pepper, julienned
- 1/2 cup mayonnaise (make sure it is low FODMAP)
- Salt and pepper to taste

Instructions:

1. Lay out the lettuce leaves and pat dry if wet.
2. Spread a thin layer of mayonnaise on each lettuce leaf.
3. Layer each leaf with the turkey slices, Swiss cheese, cucumber slices, julienned carrots, and red bell pepper.
4. Season with a sprinkle of salt and pepper to taste.
5. Carefully roll up the lettuce leaves, securing with a toothpick if necessary.
6. Serve immediately or wrap in plastic wrap and refrigerate for up to 2 hours before serving.

Nutritional Values: Calories: 350 | Carbohydrates: 8g | Protein: 33g | Fat: 20g | Fiber: 3g | Sugar: 5g

Note: For those with lactose intolerance, Swiss cheese is usually well-tolerated as it contains truly little lactose. However, if you are sensitive, you can replace the Swiss cheese with a lactose-free cheese of your choice.

Preparation time: 20 minutes | Cooking time: 40 minutes | Serves: 4

Ingredients:

- 1 medium butternut squash, peeled and cubed
- 1 tablespoon olive oil
- 1 leek (green part only), sliced
- 2 carrots, peeled and sliced
- 4 cups low-sodium vegetable broth
- Salt and pepper to taste
- A handful of fresh chives, finely chopped (for garnish)

Instructions:

1. Heat the olive oil in a large pot over medium heat.
2. Add the leek and carrots, cook until softened, about 5 minutes.
3. Add the butternut squash to the pot and stir to combine with the leek and carrots.
4. Pour in the vegetable broth and bring to a boil.
5. Once boiling, reduce the heat to low and let simmer for about 30 minutes, or until the butternut squash is soft.
6. Using a blender or immersion blender, puree the soup until smooth. If using a blender, return the soup to the pot after blending.
7. Season with salt and pepper to taste.
8. Serve hot, garnished with chopped chives.

Nutritional Values: Calories: 130 | Carbohydrates: 27g | Protein: 3g | Fat: 4g | Fiber: 6g | Sugar: 7g

Note: For those with a lactose intolerance, this recipe is naturally lactose-free.

Preparation time: 15 minutes | Cooking time: 20 minutes | Serves: 4

Ingredients:

- 1 block firm tofu, pressed and cut into cubes
- 2 tablespoons sesame oil
- 1 bell pepper, sliced
- 1 zucchini, sliced
- 1 cup canned bamboo shoots, drained
- 1 cup canned water chestnuts, drained
- 2 green onions (green parts only), sliced
- 2 tablespoons gluten-free soy sauce
- 1 tablespoon rice vinegar
- 1 tablespoon grated fresh ginger
- 2 tablespoons sesame seeds
- Cooked quinoa or rice for serving

Instructions:

1. In a large wok or frying pan, heat 1 tablespoon of sesame oil over medium heat. Add the tofu cubes and cook until golden brown on all sides, about 10 minutes. Remove from pan and set aside.
2. In the same pan, add the remaining sesame oil, bell pepper, zucchini, bamboo shoots, and water chestnuts. Stir-fry for 5-7 minutes or until the vegetables are tender-crisp.
3. While the vegetables are cooking, mix the soy sauce, rice vinegar, and grated ginger in a small bowl.
4. Add the cooked tofu back to the pan along with the soy sauce mixture. Stir well to combine and cook for another 2-3 minutes until everything is well coated and heated through.
5. Serve the stir-fry over cooked quinoa or rice, garnished with the sliced green onions and sesame seeds.

Nutritional Values: Calories: 235 | Carbohydrates: 18g | Protein: 14g | Fat: 13g | Fiber: 5g | Sugar: 6g.

Preparation time: 10 minutes | Cooking time: 15 minutes | Serves: 4

Ingredients:

- 4 halibut steaks, about 6 oz each
- Salt and pepper to taste
- 1/4 cup olive oil
- Juice and zest of 1 lemon
- 2 tablespoons chopped fresh parsley
- 2 tablespoons chopped fresh chives
- 1 tablespoon chopped fresh dill

Instructions:

1. Preheat your grill to medium heat.
2. Season the halibut steaks on both sides with salt and pepper.
3. In a small bowl, combine the olive oil, lemon juice, lemon zest, parsley, chives, and dill. Stir until well combined.
4. Brush the halibut steaks on both sides with the lemon herb sauce, reserving some for serving.
5. Grill the halibut steaks for about 5-7 minutes on each side, or until the fish flakes easily with a fork.
6. Serve the grilled halibut with the remaining lemon herb sauce drizzled on top.

Nutritional Values: Calories: 230 | Carbohydrates: 1g | Protein: 35g | Fat: 10g | Sugar: 0g

DINNER RECIPES

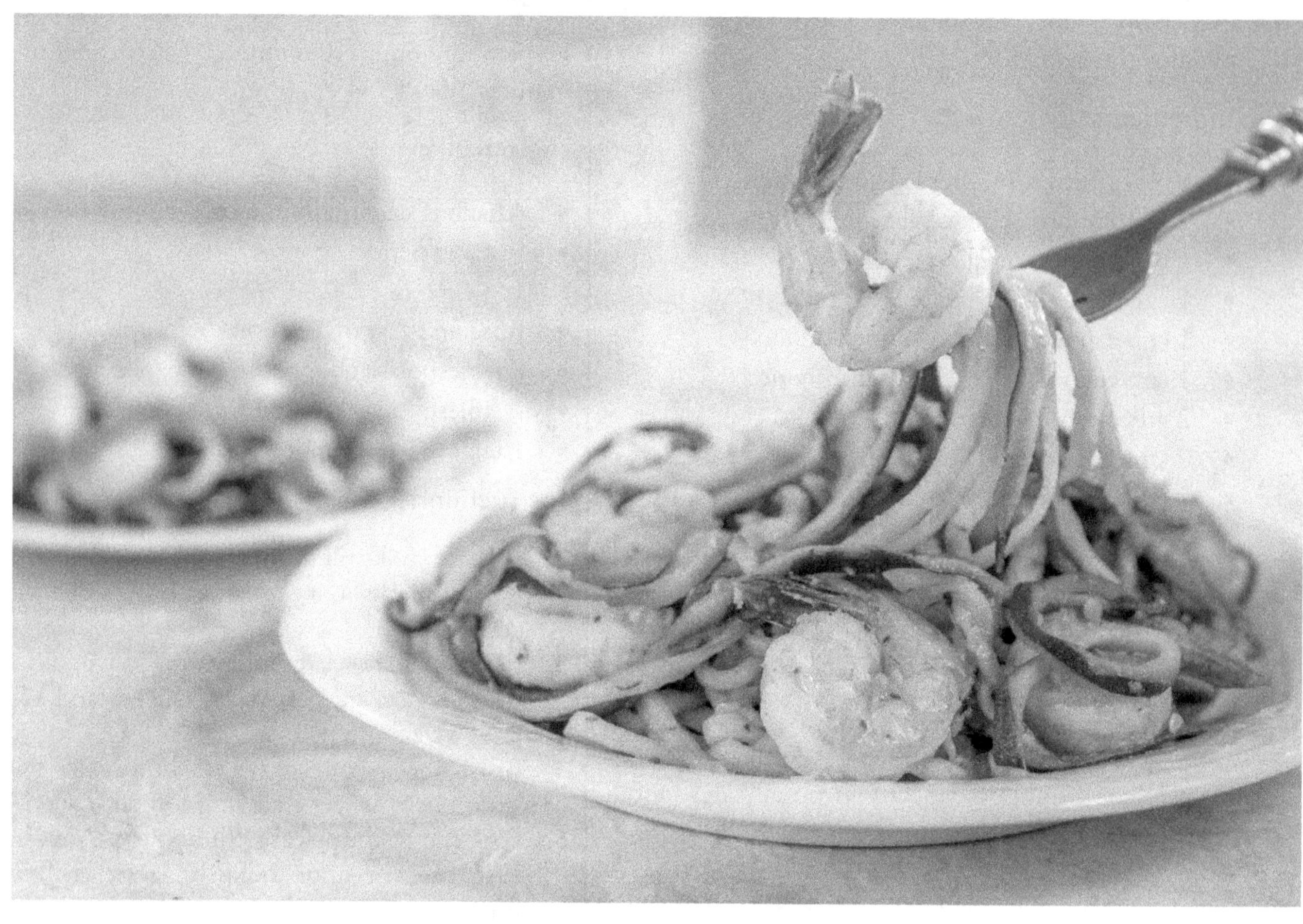

Preparation time: 10 minutes | Cooking time: 15 minutes | Servings: 4

Ingredients:

- 4 salmon fillets (about 6 ounces each)
- 2 tablespoons olive oil
- 2 lemons, zested and juiced
- 2 tablespoons fresh dill, chopped
- Salt and pepper to taste
- Lemon slices, for garnish
- Fresh dill sprigs, for garnish

Instructions:

1. Preheat your grill to medium-high heat.
2. Rinse the salmon fillets under freezing water and pat them dry with a paper towel.
3. In a small bowl, combine the olive oil, lemon zest, lemon juice, and chopped dill. Whisk until well combined.
4. Brush the salmon fillets with the lemon dill mixture and season with salt and pepper.
5. Place the salmon fillets on the grill, skin side down, and cook for 7-8 minutes. Flip the salmon over and cook for another 3-4 minutes or until cooked to your desired doneness.
6. Serve the grilled salmon fillets with additional lemon slices and sprigs of fresh dill.

Nutritional Values: Calories: 265 | Protein: 34g | Carbohydrates: 2g | Fiber: 0g | Sugars: 1g | Fat: 13g

Preparation time: 20 minutes | Cooking time: 15 minutes | Servings: 4

Ingredients:

- 4 boneless, skinless chicken breasts
- 1 cup low-FODMAP teriyaki sauce (check label for potential trigger ingredients, some brands make a gluten-free version)
- 1 small pineapple, diced
- 1 green bell pepper, diced
- 1 bunch of scallions, green parts only, thinly sliced
- 2 tablespoons rice vinegar
- 1 tablespoon sesame oil
- Salt and pepper to taste
- Wooden skewers, soaked in water for 30 minutes

Instructions:

1. Cut the chicken into bite-sized pieces. Place in a bowl and pour over the teriyaki sauce, ensuring the chicken is well coated. Marinate for at least 15 minutes.
2. While the chicken is marinating, prepare the pineapple salsa. Combine the diced pineapple, diced bell pepper, sliced scallions, rice vinegar, and sesame oil in a bowl. Stir well to combine and season with salt and pepper. Set aside.
3. Preheat your grill or grill pan to medium-high heat.
4. Thread the marinated chicken pieces onto the soaked skewers.
5. Grill the chicken skewers for 5-7 minutes on each side, or until the chicken is cooked through and has nice grill marks.
6. Serve the grilled chicken skewers with the pineapple salsa.

Nutritional Values: Calories: 280 | Protein: 26g | Carbohydrates: 24g | Fiber: 2g | Sugars: 18g | Fat: 7g

43. Garlic Infused Olive Oil Shrimp Scampi

Preparation time: 10 minutes | Cooking time: 15 minutes | Servings: 4

Ingredients:

- 1.5 lbs large shrimp, peeled and deveined
- 2 tablespoons garlic-infused olive oil
- 1/4 cup dry white wine (substitute with chicken broth for alcohol-free version)
- Zest and juice of 1 lemon
- 1 tablespoon fresh chopped parsley
- 1 tablespoon fresh chopped chives
- Salt and pepper to taste
- Lemon slices, for garnish
- 4 cups cooked gluten-free spaghetti or spiralized zucchini (zoodles), for serving

Instructions:

1. In a large skillet, heat the garlic-infused olive oil over medium heat.
2. Add the shrimp to the skillet and season with salt and pepper. Cook until the shrimp are pink and opaque, about 3-4 minutes per side.
3. Remove the shrimp from the skillet and set aside.
4. In the same skillet, add the white wine and lemon juice. Bring to a simmer and let it reduce by half, about 2-3 minutes.
5. Return the shrimp to the skillet, add the lemon zest, parsley, and chives. Stir to coat the shrimp in the sauce.
6. Serve the shrimp scampi over the cooked spaghetti or zoodles, garnish with lemon slices, and enjoy!

Nutritional Values: Calories: 320 | Protein: 32g | Carbohydrates: 30g (If served with gluten-free spaghetti) | Fiber: 2g | Sugars: 2g | Fat: 8g

44. Zucchini Noodles with Lemon Garlic Shrimp

Preparation time: 10 minutes | Cooking time: 10 minutes | Servings: 4

Ingredients:

- 4 medium zucchinis, spiralized
- 1.5 lbs large shrimp, peeled and deveined
- 2 tablespoons garlic-infused olive oil
- Zest and juice of 1 lemon
- 1/4 teaspoon red pepper flakes (optional)
- Salt and pepper to taste
- 2 tablespoons fresh chopped parsley

Instructions:

1. Heat 1 tablespoon of garlic-infused olive oil in a large skillet over medium heat.
2. Add the shrimp to the skillet, season with salt, pepper, and red pepper flakes. Cook until the shrimp are pink and opaque, about 2-3 minutes per side. Remove the shrimp from the skillet and set aside.
3. In the same skillet, add the remaining tablespoon of olive oil. Add the spiralized zucchini and cook until just tender, about 2-3 minutes.
4. Return the shrimp to the skillet, add the lemon zest and juice, and toss everything together to combine.
5. Sprinkle with fresh chopped parsley and serve immediately.

Nutritional Values: Calories: 240 | Protein: 28g | Carbohydrates: 10g | Fiber: 3g | Sugars: 6g | Fat: 10g

Preparation time: 15 minutes | Cooking time: 15 minutes | Servings: 4

Ingredients:

- 1.5 lbs lean beef, sliced into thin strips
- 2 tablespoons garlic-infused olive oil
- 2 bell peppers (red and yellow), sliced into thin strips
- 1 large zucchini, sliced into half-moons
- 1 cup Thai basil leaves
- 2 tablespoons soy sauce (ensure gluten-free)
- 1 tablespoon fish sauce
- 1 teaspoon sugar
- 1/4 teaspoon red pepper flakes (optional)
- Salt to taste

Instructions:

1. In a large skillet or wok, heat the garlic-infused olive oil over medium heat.
2. Add the beef to the skillet and cook until it is browned on all sides, about 3-5 minutes. Remove the beef from the skillet and set it aside.
3. In the same skillet, add the bell peppers and zucchini. Cook until they are tender, about 5-7 minutes.
4. Return the beef to the skillet and add the Thai basil leaves, soy sauce, fish sauce, sugar, and red pepper flakes. Stir everything together to combine.
5. Cook for another 2-3 minutes, until the basil leaves have wilted and everything is well coated in the sauce. Season with salt to taste.
6. Serve the stir fry hot, optionally over a bed of jasmine rice if tolerated.

Nutritional Values: Calories: 300 | Protein: 35g | Carbohydrates: 8g | Fiber: 2g | Sugars: 4g | Fat: 14g

Preparation time: 15 minutes | Cooking time: 1 hour 30 minutes | Servings: 6

Ingredients:

- 2 lbs pork roast (loin or shoulder)
- 2 tablespoons garlic-infused olive oil
- 1/2 cup pure maple syrup
- 1 tablespoon Dijon mustard
- 2 tablespoons apple cider vinegar
- 1 teaspoon dried thyme
- 1 teaspoon dried rosemary
- Salt and pepper to taste
- 6 large carrots, peeled and cut into 2-inch pieces

Instructions:

1. Preheat your oven to 375°F (190°C) and lightly oil a large roasting pan.
2. Season the pork roast with salt, pepper, thyme, and rosemary.
3. Heat the garlic-infused olive oil in a large skillet over medium heat. Add the pork roast and sear it on all sides until browned.
4. In a small bowl, whisk together the maple syrup, Dijon mustard, and apple cider vinegar. Pour this mixture over the seared pork roast.
5. Transfer the pork to your prepared roasting pan and arrange the carrots around it.
6. Roast in the preheated oven for about 1.5 hours, or until the pork is cooked through and the carrots are tender. Baste the pork with the pan juices every 30 minutes.
7. Let the pork rest for 10 minutes before slicing. Serve hot with the glazed carrots.

Nutritional Values: Calories: 450 | Protein: 35g | Carbohydrates: 25g | Fiber: 2g | Sugars: 20g | Fat: 20g

Preparation time: 10 minutes | Cooking time: 20 minutes | Servings: 4

Ingredients:

- 4 cod fillets (6 ounces each)
- 2 tablespoons garlic-infused olive oil
- Salt and pepper to taste
- 4 medium tomatoes, sliced
- 1/4 cup fresh basil leaves, torn
- 1 tablespoon lemon juice
- 4 tablespoons grated Parmesan cheese (Lactose intolerant individuals can substitute with lactose-free cheese or skip this ingredient)

Instructions:

1. Preheat your oven to 400°F (200°C) and lightly oil a baking dish.
2. Arrange the cod fillets in the prepared dish. Drizzle with garlic-infused olive oil, then season with salt and pepper.
3. Top each fillet with sliced tomatoes, torn basil leaves, and a sprinkle of Parmesan cheese.
4. Drizzle the lemon juice over the top of the fillets.
5. Bake in the preheated oven for 15-20 minutes, or until the fish flakes easily with a fork.
6. Serve the baked cod hot, garnished with additional fresh basil leaves if desired.

Nutritional Values: Calories: 280 | Protein: 30g | Carbohydrates: 7g | Fiber: 2g | Sugars: 4g | Fat: 14g

Preparation time: 15 minutes | Cooking time: 20 minutes | Servings: 4

Ingredients:

- 2 chicken breasts, boneless, skinless, cut into thin strips
- 1 tablespoon garlic-infused olive oil
- 1 medium red bell pepper, sliced into thin strips
- 2 medium carrots, julienned
- 1 medium zucchini, julienned
- 1 cup canned bamboo shoots, drained
- 1/4 cup low sodium soy sauce (use tamari sauce for a gluten-free option)
- 1 tablespoon cornstarch
- 1/4 cup water
- Salt and pepper to taste
- 2 green onions (green part only), chopped for garnish

Instructions:

1. Heat the garlic-infused olive oil in a large pan or wok over medium heat.
2. Add the chicken strips to the pan and stir-fry until they are no longer pink inside. Remove the cooked chicken from the pan and set it aside.
3. Add the bell pepper, carrots, zucchini, and bamboo shoots to the pan. Stir-fry the vegetables for 5-7 minutes, or until they are tender-crisp.
4. While the vegetables are cooking, whisk together the soy sauce, cornstarch, and water in a small bowl.
5. Add the cooked chicken back to the pan with the vegetables. Pour the soy sauce mixture over everything and stir well to combine.
6. Cook the stir-fry for an additional 2-3 minutes, or until the sauce has thickened.
7. Season with salt and pepper to taste.
8. Serve the stir-fry hot, garnished with chopped green onions.

Nutritional Values: Calories: 210 | Protein: 24g | Carbohydrates: 12g | Fiber: 3g | Sugars: 5g | Fat: 7g

Preparation time: 15 minutes | Cooking time: 10 minutes | Servings: 4

Ingredients:

- 4 steaks (choice cuts like ribeye, strip, or filet mignon)
- Salt and pepper to taste
- 1 cup packed fresh parsley leaves
- 1/2 cup packed fresh cilantro leaves
- 1/4 cup red wine vinegar
- 1/2 cup garlic-infused olive oil
- 1/2 teaspoon red pepper flakes (optional, for heat)
- 1/2 teaspoon ground cumin
- 1/2 teaspoon salt

Instructions:

1. Preheat your grill to high heat.
2. Season both sides of each steak with salt and pepper to taste.
3. Grill the steaks to your desired level of doneness (approximately 4-5 minutes per side for medium-rare, depending on the thickness of the steak).
4. While the steaks are grilling, make the chimichurri sauce. Combine the parsley, cilantro, red wine vinegar, garlic-infused olive oil, red pepper flakes (if using), cumin, and salt in a food processor or blender. Blend until smooth.
5. After the steaks are done grilling, let them rest for a few minutes before serving.
6. Serve each steak with a generous spoonful of chimichurri sauce on top.

Nutritional Values: Calories: 530 | Protein: 45g | Carbohydrates: 2g | Fiber: 1g | Sugars: 0g | Fat: 37g

Preparation time: 10 minutes | Cooking time: 40 minutes | Servings: 4

Ingredients:

- 8 bone-in, skin-on chicken thighs
- Salt and pepper to taste
- 1 tablespoon garlic-infused olive oil
- 2 tablespoons fresh rosemary leaves, finely chopped
- 1 tablespoon lemon zest
- 2 tablespoons lemon juice
- 1 pound carrots, peeled and cut into bite-size pieces
- 1 pound red potatoes, cut into bite-size pieces

Instructions:

1. Preheat your oven to 425°F (220°C).
2. Season both sides of each chicken thigh with salt and pepper.
3. In a small bowl, combine the garlic-infused olive oil, rosemary, lemon zest, and lemon juice. Rub this mixture all over the chicken thighs.
4. Arrange the chicken thighs in a large baking dish. Surround them with the carrots and potatoes.
5. Bake for 35-40 minutes, or until the chicken is cooked through and the vegetables are tender. If desired, broil for an additional 2-3 minutes to crisp up the chicken skin.
6. Allow the chicken to rest for a few minutes before serving.

Nutritional Values: Calories: 460 | Protein: 40g | Carbohydrates: 30g | Fiber: 5g | Sugars: 6g | Fat: 20g

Preparation time: 15 minutes | Cooking time: 35 minutes | Servings: 4

Ingredients:

- 4 large bell peppers (any color), tops cut off and seeds removed
- 1 lb lean ground beef
- 1 red bell pepper, finely chopped
- 1 medium carrot, finely chopped
- 1/2 cup quinoa, cooked
- 1 tablespoon garlic-infused olive oil
- 1 teaspoon smoked paprika
- 1 teaspoon cumin
- Salt and pepper to taste
- 1 cup low FODMAP marinara sauce
- 1/4 cup fresh chopped parsley

Instructions:

1. Preheat your oven to 375°F (190°C).
2. In a large skillet, heat the garlic-infused olive oil over medium-high heat. Add the ground beef and cook until browned and crumbly, about 5-7 minutes. Drain off any excess fat.
3. Stir in the chopped red bell pepper, carrot, cooked quinoa, paprika, and cumin. Season with salt and pepper to taste. Cook for another 5 minutes, or until the vegetables are tender.
4. Divide the beef mixture among the hollowed-out bell peppers. Place the peppers in a baking dish and cover with foil.
5. Bake for 25 minutes, then uncover and bake for another 10 minutes, or until the peppers are tender.
6. Warm the marinara sauce in a small saucepan over medium heat. Pour the sauce over the baked peppers before serving, and garnish with the chopped parsley.

Nutritional Values: Calories: 340 | Protein: 27g | Carbohydrates: 23g | Fiber: 5g | Sugars: 8g | Fat: 14g

Preparation time: 15 minutes | Cooking time: 90 minutes | Servings: 6

Ingredients:

- 1 bone-in turkey breast (about 5-6 pounds)
- 3 tablespoons garlic-infused olive oil
- Zest and juice of 1 lemon
- 1 tablespoon fresh thyme leaves, chopped
- 1 tablespoon fresh rosemary leaves, chopped
- Salt and black pepper to taste
- 1 cup low-sodium chicken broth

Instructions:

1. Preheat your oven to 350°F (175°C).
2. Rinse the turkey breast and pat dry with paper towels. Place it skin-side up in a roasting pan.
3. In a small bowl, combine the garlic-infused olive oil, lemon zest, lemon juice, thyme, and rosemary. Rub this mixture all over the turkey breast, making sure to get some under the skin.
4. Season the turkey with salt and pepper to taste.
5. Pour the chicken broth into the bottom of the roasting pan.
6. Roast the turkey in the preheated oven for about 90 minutes, or until the internal temperature reaches 165°F (74°C) when tested with a meat thermometer.
7. Let the turkey rest for 10-15 minutes before carving.

Nutritional Values: Calories: 330 | Protein: 57g | Carbohydrates: 2g | Fiber: 0g | Sugars: 1g | Fat: 11g

53. Grilled Halibut with Lemon Caper Sauce

Preparation time: 15 minutes | Cooking time: 10 minutes | Servings: 4

Ingredients:

- 4 halibut fillets (about 6 ounces each)
- Salt and pepper to taste
- 2 tablespoons garlic-infused olive oil
- 1 tablespoon lemon juice
- 1 tablespoon capers, drained
- 1 tablespoon fresh parsley, chopped
- Lemon wedges, for serving

Instructions:

1. Preheat your grill to medium-high heat.
2. Season the halibut fillets on both sides with salt and pepper.
3. Brush the grill grates with a bit of the garlic-infused olive oil, then place the halibut on the grill.
4. Cook for about 5 minutes on each side, or until the fish flakes easily with a fork.
5. While the fish is grilling, in a small bowl, mix the remaining garlic-infused olive oil, lemon juice, capers, and parsley.
6. Once the halibut is done, drizzle the lemon caper sauce over the top.
7. Serve the grilled halibut with lemon wedges on the side.

Nutritional Values: Calories: 220 | Protein: 34g | Carbohydrates: 1g | Fiber: 0g | Sugars: 0g | Fat: 9g

54. Shrimp and Pineapple Fried Rice

Preparation time: 15 minutes | Cooking time: 20 minutes | Servings: 4

Ingredients:

- 2 cups cooked basmati rice
- 1 cup shrimp, peeled and deveined
- 1 cup pineapple chunks (fresh or canned in juice, not syrup)
- 2 tablespoons garlic-infused olive oil
- 2 medium carrots, diced
- 1 red bell pepper, diced
- 2 green onions, green parts only, thinly sliced
- 2 tablespoons low sodium soy sauce (gluten-free if necessary)
- 1 tablespoon sesame oil
- Salt to taste
- Freshly ground black pepper to taste

Instructions:

1. Heat 1 tablespoon of the garlic-infused olive oil in a large skillet or wok over medium-high heat.
2. Add the shrimp and cook until they turn pink, about 2-3 minutes. Remove the shrimp from the skillet and set aside.
3. In the same skillet, add the remaining tablespoon of garlic-infused olive oil, carrots, and bell pepper. Sauté until the vegetables are tender, about 5 minutes.
4. Add the cooked rice to the skillet, stirring to mix well with the vegetables. Cook for 2-3 minutes.
5. Add the pineapple chunks, cooked shrimp, green onions, soy sauce, and sesame oil to the skillet. Stir well to combine, cooking for another 2-3 minutes until everything is well heated.
6. Season with salt and freshly ground black pepper to taste.
7. Serve hot, garnished with additional sliced green onions if desired.

Nutritional Values: Calories: 270 | Protein: 15g | Carbohydrates: 35g | Fiber: 2g | Sugars: 7g | Fat: 8g

Preparation Time: 20 minutes | Cooking Time: 40 minutes | Serves: 4

Ingredients:

- 2 medium acorn squashes
- 2 tablespoons olive oil
- Salt and pepper to taste
- 1 cup quinoa
- 2 cups vegetable broth (ensure it is low FODMAP)
- 2 cups chopped kale
- 1/4 cup chopped fresh parsley
- 1 tablespoon fresh lemon juice
- 1 tablespoon nutritional yeast
- 1/4 cup chopped walnuts

Instructions:

1. Preheat your oven to 400°F (200°C). Slice the acorn squash in half from stem to end and scoop out the seeds.
2. Brush the inside of each squash half with olive oil and season with salt and pepper. Place them on a baking sheet, cut side down, and roast for about 30 minutes or until the squash is tender and easily pierced with a fork.
3. While the squash is roasting, rinse the quinoa under icy water until the water runs clear. Place the rinsed quinoa and vegetable broth in a medium saucepan. Bring to a boil, then reduce heat to low, cover, and let simmer for 15 minutes or until all the liquid is absorbed.
4. Once the quinoa is cooked, stir in the chopped kale, parsley, lemon juice, and nutritional yeast. The heat from the quinoa will lightly cook the kale.
5. Take the squash out of the oven and flip them over. Divide the quinoa and kale stuffing evenly among the squash halves. Top with chopped walnuts.
6. Return the stuffed squash to the oven and roast for an additional 10 minutes or until the top is slightly crispy.
7. Serve and enjoy your delicious and hearty vegan meal!

Nutritional Values: Calories: 380 kcal | Carbs: 55g | Protein: 10g | Fat: 16g | Fiber: 8g | Sugar: 3g

Preparation time: 10 minutes | Cooking time: 20 minutes | Servings: 4

Ingredients:

- 4 salmon fillets
- 2 tablespoons garlic-infused olive oil
- Salt to taste
- Freshly ground black pepper to taste
- 1 lemon, zested and juiced
- 1 tablespoon fresh thyme leaves
- Lemon slices, for garnish
- Fresh thyme sprigs, for garnish

Instructions:

1. Preheat your oven to 400°F (200°C) and line a baking sheet with parchment paper.
2. Place the salmon fillets on the prepared baking sheet and drizzle with garlic-infused olive oil. Season with salt and freshly ground black pepper.
3. Sprinkle the lemon zest and fresh thyme leaves over the salmon fillets.
4. Drizzle the lemon juice evenly over the salmon fillets.
5. Place the baking sheet in the oven and bake for 15-20 minutes, or until the salmon is cooked through and flakes easily with a fork.
6. Serve the salmon hot, garnished with fresh thyme sprigs and lemon slices.

Nutritional Values: Calories: 320 | Protein: 35g | Carbohydrates: 2g | Fiber: 1g | Sugars: 1g | Fat: 20g

Preparation time: 15 minutes | **Cooking time:** 45 minutes | **Servings:** 4

Ingredients:

- 1 medium spaghetti squash
- 2 tablespoons garlic-infused olive oil
- Salt to taste
- Freshly ground black pepper to taste
- 1 can (400g) diced tomatoes, no onion or garlic added
- 1/4 cup fresh basil, finely chopped
- 1 teaspoon dried oregano
- 1 tablespoon balsamic vinegar
- Grated Parmesan cheese, for serving (optional, remove for vegan option)

Instructions:

1. Preheat your oven to 400°F (200°C) and line a baking sheet with parchment paper.
2. Cut the spaghetti squash in half lengthwise and scoop out the seeds.
3. Drizzle the inside of the squash with 1 tablespoon of garlic-infused olive oil and season with salt and pepper.
4. Place the squash cut side down on the prepared baking sheet and bake for about 35-40 minutes, or until the squash is tender and easily shreds with a fork.
5. While the squash is cooking, prepare the sauce by heating the remaining olive oil in a pan over medium heat.
6. Add the diced tomatoes, basil, oregano, and balsamic vinegar. Simmer for 20-25 minutes, or until the sauce has thickened.
7. Once the squash is cooked, use a fork to shred the squash into spaghetti-like strands.
8. Serve the spaghetti squash with the tomato basil sauce on top, garnished with a sprinkling of Parmesan cheese if desired.

Nutritional Values: Calories: 170 | Protein: 3g | Carbohydrates: 20g | Fiber: 4g | Sugars: 7g | Fat: 10g

Note: For a vegan version, simply omit the Parmesan cheese or use a vegan alternative.

Preparation time: 20 minutes | **Cooking time:** 40 minutes | **Servings:** 4

Ingredients:

- 1 large eggplant, diced
- 2 medium zucchinis, diced
- 1 red bell pepper, diced
- 1 green bell pepper, diced
- 2 tablespoons garlic-infused olive oil
- 1 can (400g) diced tomatoes, no onion or garlic added
- 1 teaspoon dried thyme
- 1 teaspoon dried rosemary
- Salt to taste
- Freshly ground black pepper to taste
- Fresh basil leaves for garnish

Instructions:

1. Heat the garlic-infused olive oil in a large pan over medium heat.
2. Add the diced eggplant, zucchinis, and bell peppers to the pan. Cook for about 10 minutes, or until the vegetables begin to soften.
3. Add the diced tomatoes, thyme, rosemary, salt, and pepper to the pan. Stir to combine.
4. Reduce the heat to low, cover the pan, and let the mixture simmer for about 30 minutes, or until the vegetables are completely tender.
5. Check the seasoning and adjust if necessary. Garnish with fresh basil leaves before serving.

Nutritional Values: Calories: 140 | Protein: 3g | Carbohydrates: 17g | Fiber: 7g | Sugars: 10g | Fat: 8g

59. Rainbow Quinoa Salad with Lemon Vinaigrette (VG)

Preparation time: 15 minutes | Cooking time: 20 minutes | Servings: 4

Ingredients:

- 1 cup uncooked quinoa
- 2 cups water
- 1 small red bell pepper, diced
- 1 small yellow bell pepper, diced
- 1 small cucumber, diced
- 1/2 cup cherry tomatoes, halved
- 1/4 cup fresh chopped parsley
- 1/4 cup fresh chopped mint
- 2 tablespoons garlic-infused olive oil
- Juice of 1 lemon
- Salt to taste
- Freshly ground black pepper to taste

Instructions:

1. Rinse the quinoa under cold water until the water runs clear. Add the quinoa and water to a medium saucepan, then bring to a boil over high heat. Reduce the heat to low, cover, and let the quinoa simmer for 15 minutes, or until all the water is absorbed.
2. While the quinoa is cooking, prepare the vegetables. In a large bowl, combine the bell peppers, cucumber, cherry tomatoes, parsley, and mint.
3. In a separate small bowl, whisk together the garlic-infused olive oil, lemon juice, salt, and pepper to create the vinaigrette.
4. Once the quinoa is cooked, fluff it with a fork and let it cool for a few minutes. Then add the quinoa to the bowl with the vegetables.
5. Drizzle the vinaigrette over the quinoa and vegetables, then toss everything together until well combined. Serve the salad chilled or at room temperature.

Nutritional Values: Calories: 245 | Protein: 7g | Carbohydrates: 35g | Fiber: 5g | Sugars: 4g | Fat: 9g

60. Stir-Fried Tofu with Bell Peppers and Broccoli (VG)

Preparation time: 15 minutes | Cooking time: 15 minutes | Servings: 4

Ingredients:

- 1 block (14 ounces) firm tofu
- 2 tablespoons garlic-infused olive oil
- 1 large red bell pepper, thinly sliced
- 1 large green bell pepper, thinly sliced
- 2 tablespoons low-sodium soy sauce or tamari for gluten-free
- 1 tablespoon rice vinegar
- 1 tablespoon maple syrup
- Salt to taste
- Freshly ground black pepper to taste
- 2 tablespoons chopped fresh chives for garnish

Instructions:

1. Drain the tofu and pat it dry with paper towels. Cut the tofu into 1-inch cubes.
2. Heat 1 tablespoon of the garlic-infused olive oil in a large skillet or wok over medium-high heat. Add the tofu cubes and cook until they are browned on all sides, about 7-8 minutes. Remove the tofu from the skillet and set it aside.
3. In the same skillet, heat the remaining olive oil. Add the bell peppers and stir-fry for about 5 minutes, or until they are tender-crisp.
4. In a small bowl, whisk together the soy sauce or tamari, rice vinegar, and maple syrup. Pour this mixture into the skillet with the bell peppers.
5. Return the tofu to the skillet, stirring to coat it with the sauce and to heat it through.
6. Season with salt and pepper to taste. Garnish with fresh chives before serving.

Nutritional Values: Calories: 215 | Protein: 13g | Carbohydrates: 15g | Fiber: 3g | Sugars: 7g | Fat: 12g

Note: Please note that many soy sauces contain wheat, which can be a problem for people with gluten intolerance, so it is better to opt for tamari which is normally gluten-free.

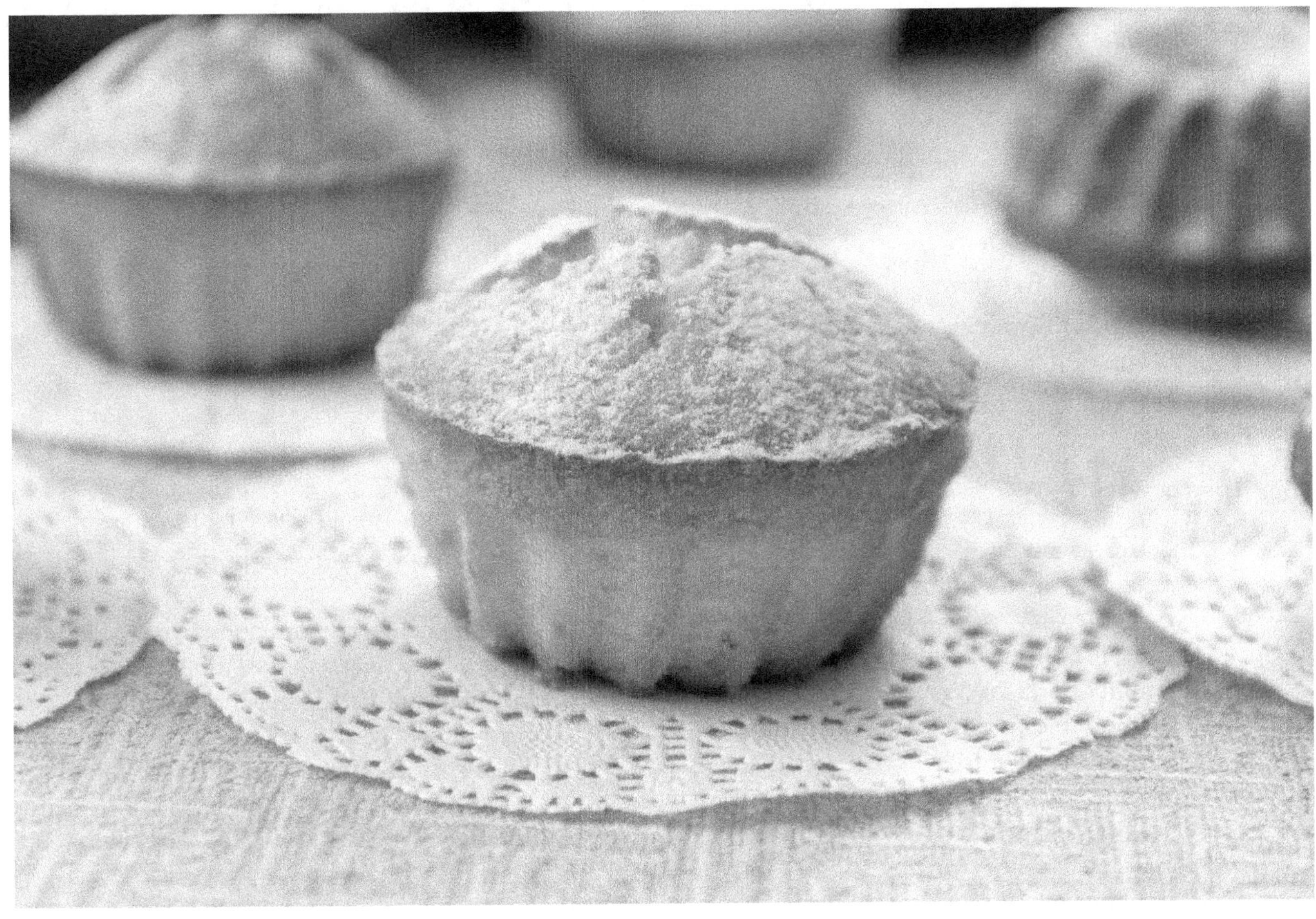

61. Chia Seed and Blueberry Energy Balls (VG)

Preparation Time: 15 minutes | Cooking Time: 0 minutes | Portion Size: Makes 12 balls

Ingredients:

- 1 cup blueberries (frozen or fresh)
- 1/2 cup chia seeds
- 1 cup gluten-free oats
- 1/2 cup sunflower seeds
- 1/4 cup pure maple syrup
- 1/2 cup unsweetened shredded coconut for rolling

Instructions:

1. In a food processor, combine the blueberries, chia seeds, oats, sunflower seeds, and maple syrup.
2. Process until the mixture comes together, about 1-2 minutes.
3. Using a tablespoon, scoop out portions of the mixture and roll into balls.
4. Roll each ball in shredded coconut until coated.
5. Place the balls onto a baking sheet lined with parchment paper.
6. Refrigerate for 1 hour or until firm.
7. Store in an airtight container in the refrigerator for up to one week.

Nutritional Values: Calories: 110 | Fat: 4g | Carbohydrates: 17g | Fiber: 4g | Sugar: 8g | Protein: 3g

Note: Chia seeds are high in fiber and can absorb up to 10 times their weight in liquid, making them an excellent choice for a filling snack. Always check labels on packaged foods like oats and shredded coconut to ensure they are free of high FODMAP ingredients.

62. Baked Feta with Cherry Tomatoes (V)

Preparation time: 10 minutes | Cooking time: 20 minutes | Serving size: 4 servings

Ingredients:

- 1 block of feta cheese (200g)
- 1 cup cherry tomatoes, halved
- 2 tbsp olive oil
- 1 tsp dried oregano
- 1 tsp dried basil
- A handful of fresh basil leaves for garnish
- Salt and pepper to taste

Instructions:

1. Preheat the oven to 375°F (190°C).
2. Place the block of feta in the middle of a baking dish.
3. Scatter the cherry tomatoes around the feta.
4. Drizzle the olive oil over the feta and tomatoes.
5. Sprinkle the dried oregano, dried basil, salt, and pepper evenly over everything.
6. Bake for 20 minutes, or until the feta is soft and slightly golden on top, and the tomatoes are roasted.
7. Garnish with fresh basil leaves.
8. Serve warm with low FODMAP, gluten-free crackers or bread.

Nutritional Values: Calories: 200 | Carbs: 5g | Protein: 8g | Fat: 16g | Fiber: 1g | Sugar: 3g

Note: Please note that feta cheese is a lactose-containing food. However, hard cheeses like feta are low in lactose and are usually well tolerated by most people with lactose intolerance. If you are particularly sensitive to lactose, you may want to avoid this recipe or replace the feta cheese with a lactose-free cheese alternative.

63. FODMAP-friendly Lemon Poppy Seed Muffins

Preparation time: 15 minutes | Cooking time: 20 minutes | Serving size: 12 muffins

Ingredients:

- 2 cups gluten-free flour blend
- 1 cup granulated sugar
- 2 teaspoons baking powder
- 1/4 teaspoon salt
- 1 tablespoon poppy seeds
- 2/3 cup lactose-free milk (or almond milk for lactose intolerance)
- 1/2 cup vegetable oil
- 2 large eggs
- Zest of 2 lemons
- Juice of 2 lemons
- 1 teaspoon pure vanilla extract

Instructions:

1. Preheat the oven to 375°F (190°C) and line a muffin tin with paper liners.
2. In a large bowl, whisk together the gluten-free flour blend, sugar, baking powder, salt, and poppy seeds.
3. In a separate bowl, combine the lactose-free milk, vegetable oil, eggs, lemon zest, lemon juice, and vanilla extract. Stir until well combined.
4. Gradually add the wet ingredients to the dry ingredients, stirring just until combined. Be careful not to overmix.
5. Divide the batter evenly among the muffin cups, filling each about 2/3 full.
6. Bake for 18-20 minutes, or until a toothpick inserted into the center of a muffin comes out clean.
7. Allow the muffins to cool in the tin for 5 minutes, then transfer to a wire rack to cool completely.

Nutritional Values: Calories: 210 | Carbs: 28g | Protein: 3g | Fat: 10g | Fiber: 1g | Sugar: 14g

Note: Please note that these muffins contain eggs. If you are allergic to eggs, you can substitute them with a flax egg (1 tablespoon ground flaxseed mixed with 2.5 tablespoons water for each egg). Allow the mixture to sit for a few minutes before using.

64. Smoky Quinoa-Stuffed Mini Bell Peppers (VG)

Preparation time: 20 minutes | Cooking time: 15 minutes | Serving size: 4 servings

Ingredients:

- 16 mini bell peppers
- 1 cup cooked quinoa
- 1 can (15 oz) black beans, drained and rinsed
- 1 teaspoon smoked paprika
- 1 teaspoon ground cumin
- Salt and black pepper to taste
- 2 tablespoons olive oil
- 2 tablespoons chopped fresh cilantro
- 1 lime, juiced

Instructions:

1. Preheat your oven to 375°F (190°C) and line a baking tray with parchment paper.
2. Cut off the tops of the mini bell peppers and scoop out the seeds inside. Set aside.
3. In a large bowl, combine the cooked quinoa, drained black beans, smoked paprika, cumin, salt, and pepper. Stir until well combined.
4. Using a small spoon, stuff each mini bell pepper with the quinoa mixture. Place the stuffed peppers onto the prepared baking tray.
5. Drizzle the peppers with olive oil and bake in the preheated oven for 15 minutes, or until the peppers are tender and the filling is heated through.
6. Remove from the oven and drizzle with fresh lime juice. Garnish with chopped cilantro before serving.

Nutritional Values: Calories: 200 | Carbs: 28g | Protein: 8g | Fat: 7g | Fiber: 6g | Sugar: 4g

Note: Please note that quinoa is a naturally gluten-free grain, but if you have a gluten sensitivity, make sure the quinoa you purchase is labeled as gluten-free to avoid potential cross-contamination.

65. Quick and Easy Carrot and Cucumber Sticks with Homemade Hummus (V)

Preparation time: 10 minutes | Cooking time: 0 minutes | Serving size: 4 servings

Ingredients:

- 2 large carrots
- 1 cucumber
- 1 can (15 oz) of canned chickpeas, drained and rinsed
- 2 tablespoons tahini (sesame paste)
- 2 tablespoons garlic-infused olive oil
- Juice of 1 lemon
- Salt and pepper to taste
- 1 tablespoon chopped fresh parsley for garnish (optional)

Instructions:

1. Peel and cut the carrots and cucumber into sticks. Set aside.
2. In a food processor, combine the drained chickpeas, tahini, garlic-infused olive oil, and lemon juice. Blend until smooth.
3. Season the hummus with salt and pepper to taste, adjusting as needed.
4. Transfer the hummus to a serving bowl and garnish with chopped fresh parsley, if using.
5. Serve the carrot and cucumber sticks with the homemade hummus.

Nutritional Values: Calories: 190 | Carbs: 21g | Protein: 6g | Fat: 9g | Fiber: 6g | Sugar: 5g

Note: This recipe uses garlic-infused olive oil instead of raw garlic to keep it FODMAP-friendly. The FODMAPs in garlic are not oil-soluble, meaning you can enjoy the flavor without the potential digestive discomfort. Make sure to choose a garlic-infused oil that does not contain any actual garlic pieces, as these could still contain FODMAPs.

66. Crispy Baked Chicken Tenders with Garlic Infused Olive Oil Dipping Sauce

Preparation time: 15 minutes | Cooking time: 20 minutes | Serving size: 4 servings

Ingredients:

- 1 lb chicken tenders
- 2 cups gluten-free breadcrumbs
- 2 eggs
- 1 tablespoon dried Italian herbs
- Salt and pepper to taste
- Cooking spray
- 1/2 cup garlic-infused olive oil
- Juice of 1 lemon

Instructions:

1. Preheat your oven to 400°F (200°C) and line a baking sheet with parchment paper.
2. In a shallow bowl, beat the eggs. In another shallow bowl, combine the gluten-free breadcrumbs, dried Italian herbs, salt, and pepper.
3. Dip each chicken tender into the beaten eggs, then roll in the breadcrumb mixture. Make sure each tender is fully coated.
4. Place the breaded chicken tenders on the prepared baking sheet. Spray a light coating of cooking spray on the chicken to help it brown in the oven.
5. Bake for 15-20 minutes, or until the chicken is cooked through and the breadcrumbs are golden brown.
6. While the chicken is baking, mix the garlic-infused olive oil and lemon juice in a small bowl to make the dipping sauce.
7. Serve the baked chicken tenders hot with the garlic-infused olive oil dipping sauce on the side.

Nutritional Values: Calories: 500 | Carbs: 45g | Protein: 30g | Fat: 20g | Fiber: 2g | Sugar: 2g

Note: Garlic-infused olive oil is used to bring a garlic flavor to the dish without triggering FODMAPs, as the FODMAPs in garlic are not oil-soluble. Also, make sure that the gluten-free breadcrumbs you use do not contain any high FODMAP ingredients. This dish is a great snack or meal that everyone can enjoy.

67. Smashed Avocado on Gluten-Free Toast (V)

Preparation time: 5 minutes | Cooking time: 5 minutes | Serving size: 2 servings

Ingredients:

- 2 slices of gluten-free bread
- 1 medium ripe avocado
- Salt and pepper to taste
- A squeeze of lemon juice
- A handful of cherry tomatoes
- A pinch of red pepper flakes (optional)
- A sprinkle of chia seeds (optional)

Instructions:

1. Toast your gluten-free bread slices to your desired level of crispness.
2. While the bread is toasting, cut the avocado in half, remove the pit, and scoop out the flesh into a bowl. Mash it with a fork until it is as smooth or chunky as you like.
3. Season the mashed avocado with a pinch of salt, pepper, and a squeeze of lemon juice. Mix well.
4. Once the bread is toasted, spread the mashed avocado evenly on each slice.
5. Top each toast slice with a few cherry tomatoes, a sprinkle of red pepper flakes (if using), and chia seeds (if using).
6. Serve immediately and enjoy this refreshing and healthy snack or light meal.

Nutritional Values: Calories: 210 | Carbs: 23g | Protein: 5g | Fat: 12g | Fiber: 8g | Sugar: 3g

Note: As avocados are well tolerated in insignificant amounts by those following a low FODMAP diet, it is important to not consume too much. It is usually recommended to limit your serving to a quarter of a medium avocado. Also, make sure that the gluten-free bread you use does not contain any high FODMAP ingredients. This dish is a great light meal or snack for anyone following a low FODMAP diet.

68. Sweet Potato Fries with Paprika and Oregano

Preparation time: 10 minutes | Cooking time: 30 minutes | Serving size: 2 servings

Ingredients:

- 2 medium sweet potatoes
- 2 tablespoons olive oil
- 1 teaspoon dried oregano
- 1 teaspoon paprika
- Salt and black pepper to taste

Instructions:

1. Preheat your oven to 200°C (400°F) and line a baking tray with baking paper.
2. Wash and dry the sweet potatoes. Cut them into fries' shape, keeping the skin on for extra fiber.
3. In a large bowl, toss the sweet potato fries with olive oil, oregano, paprika, salt, and pepper until evenly coated.
4. Spread the fries out on the prepared baking tray in a single layer, making sure they do not overlap.
5. Bake for about 30 minutes, flipping halfway through, until the fries are crispy and golden brown.
6. Let the fries cool slightly before serving. These make a perfect snack or side dish.

Nutritional Values: Calories: 245 | Carbs: 32g | Protein: 2g | Fat: 12g | Fiber: 5g | Sugar: 6g

Note: Sweet potatoes are considered low FODMAP at a serving size of up to 70g (about 1/2 cup). Although sweet potatoes contain some FODMAPs, they are well tolerated when consumed in moderation. So please adjust the serving size based on your tolerance.

69. STRAWBERRY AND BANANA SMOOTHIE BOWL (VG)

Preparation time: 10 minutes | Cooking time: 0 minutes | Serving size: 1 serving

Ingredients:

- 10 small strawberries
- 1 small ripe banana
- 1/2 cup lactose-free yogurt or coconut yogurt for a vegan version
- 1 tablespoon chia seeds
- 1 tablespoon shredded coconut
- A handful of low FODMAP granola for topping
- A few fresh mint leaves for garnish (optional)

Instructions:

1. Wash the strawberries and remove the stems. Peel the banana.
2. In a blender, combine strawberries, banana, and lactose-free yogurt. Blend until smooth.
3. Pour the smoothie into a bowl.
4. Sprinkle the chia seeds, shredded coconut, and granola on top of the smoothie. You can arrange them in rows or simply sprinkle them over the smoothie.
5. Garnish with a few fresh mint leaves if desired.
6. Enjoy your low FODMAP smoothie bowl immediately for the best taste and texture.

Nutritional Values: Calories: 310 | Carbs: 53g | Protein: 11g | Fat: 8g | Fiber: 9g | Sugar: 29g

Note: Strawberries and bananas are low in FODMAPs and well tolerated by most people. However, it is always important to listen to your body and adjust serving sizes to suit your personal tolerances. Also, make sure your granola is low FODMAP - look for one that is made with oats and sweetened with maple syrup or another low FODMAP sweetener, and does not contain high FODMAP nuts like cashews or pistachios.

70. OVEN-BAKED ZUCCHINI CHIPS WITH DILL DIP (V)

Preparation time: 15 minutes | Cooking time: 25 minutes | Serving size: 4 servings

Ingredients:

- 2 medium zucchinis
- 1 cup gluten-free breadcrumbs
- 1/2 cup grated Parmesan cheese (use nutritional yeast for a vegan version)
- 1/2 teaspoon paprika
- 1/2 teaspoon garlic-infused olive oil
- Salt and pepper to taste
- 2 eggs (use plant-based milk for a vegan version)

For the Dill Dip:

- 1/2 cup lactose-free yogurt or coconut yogurt for a vegan version
- 1 tablespoon fresh dill, finely chopped
- Salt and pepper to taste

Instructions:

1. Preheat your oven to 425°F (220°C) and line a baking sheet with parchment paper.
2. Slice zucchinis into thin rounds, about 1/4 inch thick.
3. In a shallow bowl, mix gluten-free breadcrumbs, Parmesan cheese (or nutritional yeast), paprika, salt, and pepper.
4. In a separate bowl, whisk the eggs (or plant-based milk).
5. Dip each zucchini slice into the egg (or milk), then coat in the bread crumb mixture. Place on the prepared baking sheet.
6. Bake for 20-25 minutes, until golden and crisp.
7. While the zucchini chips are baking, prepare the dill dip by combining lactose-free yogurt (or coconut yogurt), dill, salt, and pepper in a small bowl.
8. Once the zucchini chips are done, serve them warm with the dill dip.

Nutrition Values: Calories: 180 | Carbs: 22g | Protein: 10g | Fat: 6g | Fiber: 2g | Sugar: 5g

Note: Make sure your breadcrumbs are made from a gluten-free grain like rice or corn, and that they do not contain any high FODMAP ingredients like onion or garlic powder. You can also make your own by toasting gluten-free bread and grinding it in a food processor. Also, ensure the yogurt is lactose-free or a non-dairy version like coconut yogurt to stay within FODMAP guidelines.

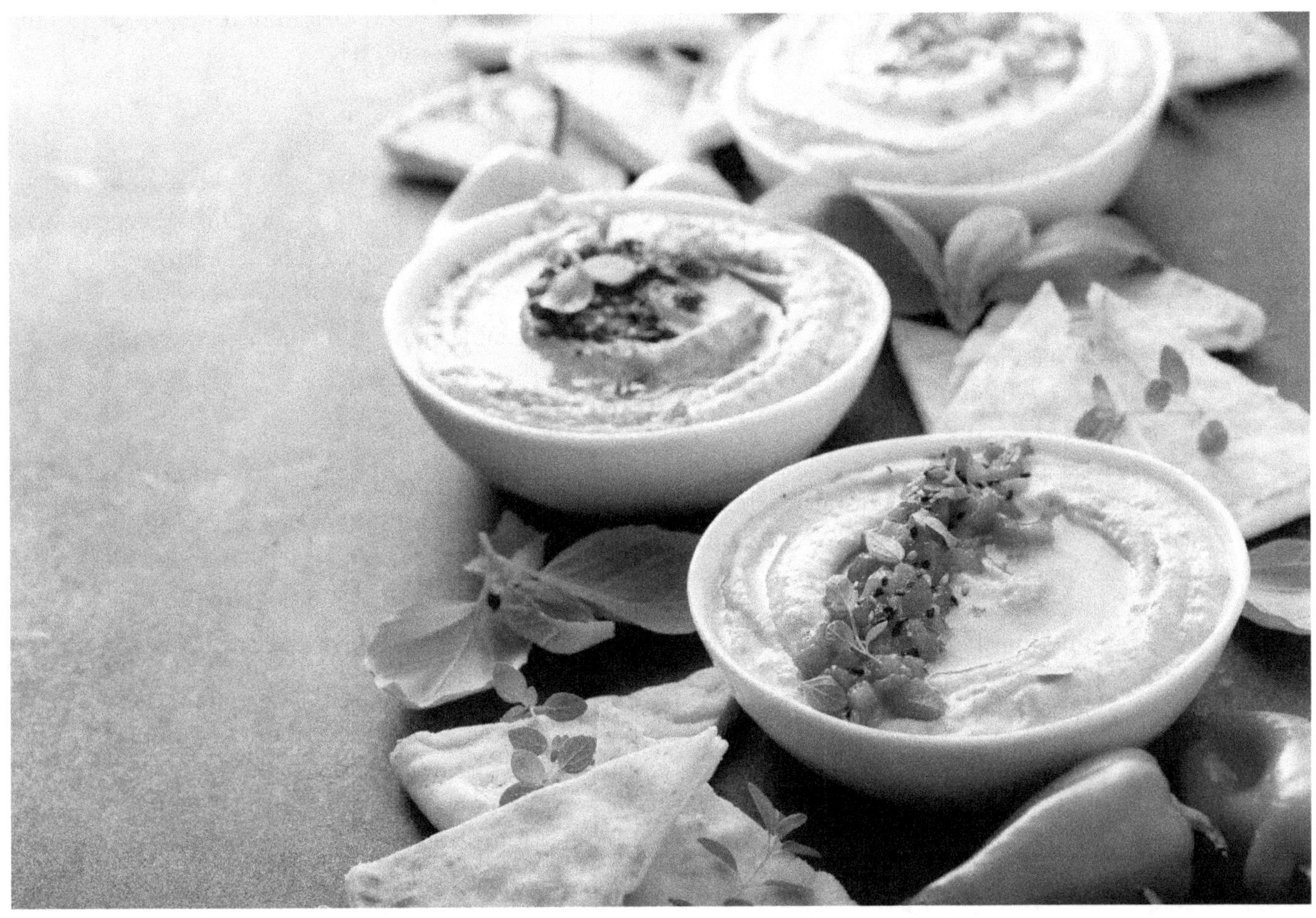

Preparation time: 5 minutes | Cooking time: 25 minutes | Makes about 1 cup

Ingredients:

- 1 cup extra-virgin olive oil
- 3 cloves of garlic (note: garlic will be removed after infusing)

Instructions:

1. Peel the garlic cloves and gently crush them with the side of a knife.
2. In a small saucepan, combine the olive oil and the crushed garlic cloves.
3. Heat the oil on low heat until it reaches a gentle simmer. Simmer for about 20-25 minutes. Make sure the garlic does not brown. If it starts to brown, lower the heat.
4. After simmering, remove the pan from heat and let the oil cool down completely.
5. Once cool, strain the oil to remove the garlic cloves and pour the oil into a clean glass jar or bottle.
6. You can use this garlic-infused olive oil immediately or store it in a cool, dark place for up to 1 month.

Nutritional Values: Calories: 120 | Fat: 14g | Carbohydrate: 0g | Fiber: 0g | Protein: 0g

Note: Garlic is a high FODMAP food, but when it is used to infuse oil, the FODMAPs (which are not oil-soluble) do not leach into the oil, making it safe for a low FODMAP diet. However, the garlic cloves themselves remain high in FODMAPs and should not be consumed.

Preparation time: 10 minutes | Cooking time: 20 minutes | Serves 4

Ingredients:

- 1 cup quinoa
- 2 cups water or low-FODMAP vegetable broth
- 1/2 cup chopped fresh cilantro
- Zest and juice of 1 lime
- 1 tablespoon garlic-infused olive oil
- Salt to taste

Instructions:

1. Rinse quinoa under icy water using a fine mesh strainer until the water runs clear.
2. Combine the rinsed quinoa and water (or vegetable broth) in a medium saucepan and bring to a boil over high heat.
3. Once boiling, reduce the heat to low, cover, and let it simmer until the quinoa is tender and the liquid is absorbed, about 15 minutes.
4. Remove from heat and let the quinoa rest, covered, for 5 minutes.
5. Fluff the quinoa with a fork, then mix in the cilantro, lime zest, lime juice, garlic-infused olive oil, and salt to taste.
6. Serve immediately or store in an airtight container in the refrigerator for up to 3 days.

Nutritional Values: Calories: 205 | Fat: 5g | Carbohydrates: 34g | Fiber: 4g | Protein: 8g

Preparation time: 10 minutes | Cooking time: 25 minutes | Serves 4

Ingredients:

- 1 pound carrots, peeled and sliced into 1/2 inch pieces
- 2 tablespoons garlic-infused olive oil
- Zest and juice of 1 lemon
- 1 teaspoon dried thyme
- 1 teaspoon dried rosemary
- Salt and pepper to taste
- Fresh parsley for garnish (optional)

Instructions:

1. Preheat your oven to 400°F (200°C) and line a baking tray with parchment paper.
2. In a large bowl, combine the sliced carrots, garlic-infused olive oil, lemon zest, lemon juice, thyme, rosemary, salt, and pepper.
3. Spread the carrots out in a single layer on the prepared baking tray.
4. Roast for 25-30 minutes, or until the carrots are tender and slightly caramelized, stirring halfway through.
5. Remove from the oven and let them cool slightly before serving. If desired, garnish with fresh parsley.

Nutritional Values: Calories: 110 | Fat: 7g | Saturated Fat: 1g | Sodium: 90mg | Carbohydrates: 12g | Fiber: 3g | Sugar: 5g | Protein: 1g

Preparation time: 10 minutes | Cooking time: 10 minutes | Serves 4

Ingredients:

- 2 medium zucchinis
- 1 tablespoon olive oil
- Zest of 1 lemon
- 1/2 teaspoon coarse sea salt
- Freshly ground black pepper

Instructions:

1. Preheat your grill to medium-high heat.
2. Slice the zucchinis lengthwise into 1/4 inch thick strips.
3. In a small bowl, mix the olive oil, lemon zest, sea salt, and a few grinds of black pepper.
4. Brush the zucchini slices on both sides with the olive oil mixture.
5. Grill the zucchini for about 4 minutes on each side, or until they have nice grill marks and are tender.
6. Serve the grilled zucchini hot, sprinkled with any remaining lemon salt.

Nutritional Values: Calories: 70 | Fat: 4g | Carbohydrates: 7g | Fiber: 2g | Sugar: 4g | Protein: 2g

Preparation time: 10 minutes | Cooking time: 30 minutes | Serves: 8

Ingredients:

- 2 cups of low FODMAP chicken broth
- 1 cup of water
- 1/4 cup of garlic-infused oil
- 1/4 cup of gluten-free flour
- 1 teaspoon of salt
- 1/2 teaspoon of freshly ground black pepper

Instructions:

1. In a large saucepan, heat the garlic-infused oil over medium heat.
2. Sprinkle the flour into the oil, stirring constantly for about 2 minutes to make a roux. It should be a light golden color.
3. Gradually whisk in the chicken broth and water, ensuring no lumps form.
4. Bring the mixture to a boil, then reduce heat and let simmer, stirring occasionally until the gravy has thickened, about 20 minutes.
5. Add salt and freshly ground black pepper, adjusting to taste.
6. Once your gravy has reached the desired thickness, remove it from heat. If you would like it smoother, you can strain it through a fine-mesh sieve.

Nutritional Values: Calories: 80 | Fat: 5g | Carbohydrates: 7g | Fiber: 0g | Sugar: 0g | Protein: 1g

Preparation time: 10 minutes | Cooking time: 20 minutes | Serves: 6

Ingredients:

- 3 large red bell peppers
- 1 tablespoon garlic-infused olive oil
- 1 cup of canned chickpeas, rinsed and drained
- 1/4 cup of tahini
- 2 tablespoons of lemon juice
- Salt and pepper to taste
- A pinch of smoked paprika (optional)

Instructions:

1. Preheat your oven to 450°F (230°C) and line a baking tray with aluminum foil.
2. Place the bell peppers on the tray and roast for about 20 minutes, or until the skin is charred and blistered. Flip the peppers halfway through to ensure they roast evenly.
3. Remove the peppers from the oven and let them cool slightly. Once they are cool enough to manage, peel off the skin and remove the seeds and stem.
4. In a food processor, combine the roasted peppers, chickpeas, tahini, lemon juice, and garlic-infused olive oil. Blend until smooth.
5. Season with salt, pepper, and smoked paprika (if using), then blend again to combine.
6. Serve the dip with gluten-free bread or low FODMAP vegetables. Store any leftovers in an airtight container in the fridge for up to a week.

Nutritional Values: Calories: 125 | Fat: 7g | Carbohydrates: 13g | Fiber: 4g | Sugar: 3g | Protein: 4g

Preparation time: 10 minutes | Cooking time: 25 minutes | Serves: 4

Ingredients:

- 1 lb fresh Brussels sprouts, halved
- 2 tablespoons olive oil
- Salt and pepper to taste
- 2 tablespoons pure maple syrup
- 1 tablespoon Dijon mustard
- 1 teaspoon apple cider vinegar

Instructions:

1. Preheat your oven to 400°F (200°C) and line a baking sheet with parchment paper.
2. Toss the halved Brussels sprouts with olive oil, salt, and pepper. Spread them out on the baking sheet in a single layer.
3. Roast the Brussels sprouts for about 20-25 minutes, or until they are tender and lightly charred.
4. While the Brussels sprouts are roasting, combine the maple syrup, Dijon mustard, and apple cider vinegar in a small bowl. Stir well to create your glaze.
5. Once the Brussels sprouts are roasted, remove them from the oven and drizzle the glaze over them. Toss well to ensure all the Brussels sprouts are coated.
6. Serve immediately while hot. Enjoy this delicious side dish that is full of flavor and fits well into a low FODMAP diet!

Nutritional Values: Calories: 150 | Fat: 7g | Carbohydrates: 20g | Fiber: 4g | Sugar: 9g | Protein: 4g

Note: Brussels sprouts are considered low FODMAP at a serving size of 38g (or about two sprouts). This recipe should be suitable for those following a low FODMAP diet, but as always, please adjust portion sizes based on your individual tolerance.

Preparation time: 15 minutes | Cooking time: 35 minutes | Serves: 4

Ingredients:

- 4 large red potatoes
- 3 tablespoons olive oil
- 2 tablespoons fresh rosemary, finely chopped
- Salt and pepper to taste
- 1 teaspoon garlic-infused oil (ensure no garlic pieces in oil)

Instructions:

1. Preheat your oven to 400°F (200°C) and line a baking tray with baking paper.
2. Clean and cut the potatoes into wedge shapes. Ensure the pieces are similar in size for even cooking.
3. In a large bowl, mix the olive oil, rosemary, salt, pepper, and garlic-infused oil.
4. Add the potato wedges to the bowl and toss until well coated.
5. Arrange the potato wedges on the prepared baking tray in a single layer.
6. Roast for 35-40 minutes or until the potatoes are golden and crispy. Halfway through, flip the potatoes to ensure they cook evenly.
7. Serve the rosemary-infused potato wedges hot. Enjoy this hearty and flavorful side dish!

Nutritional Values: Calories: 220 | Fat: 9g | Carbohydrates: 32g | Fiber: 3g | Sugar: 2g | Protein: 4g

Note: Garlic-infused oil is considered low FODMAP as the FODMAPs in garlic are not soluble in oil. Make sure to choose an oil without any pieces of garlic in it to keep this recipe FODMAP-friendly. As always, adjust portion sizes based on your individual tolerance.

Preparation time: 15 minutes | Cooking time: 3 hours | Makes: About 3 liters

Ingredients:

- 2 kg beef bones
- 2 carrots, chopped
- 1 parsnip, chopped
- 1 bunch green onions (green parts only)
- 2 tomatoes, quartered
- 2 sprigs of thyme
- 2 bay leaves
- Salt and pepper to taste
- 3 liters of water

Instructions:

1. Preheat your oven to 400°F (200°C) and place the beef bones on a baking sheet. Roast for about 30 minutes or until well browned.
2. In a large pot, add the roasted beef bones, chopped carrots, parsnip, green onion tops, quartered tomatoes, thyme, bay leaves, and seasoning. Cover with water.
3. Bring to a boil, then reduce heat and let it simmer for about 3 hours.
4. Strain the broth through a fine mesh strainer and discard the solids. Allow the broth to cool before storing.
5. Store in airtight containers in the refrigerator for up to a week or freeze for up to 3 months.

Nutritional Values: Calories: 20 | Fat: 0g | Carbohydrates: 2g | Fiber: 1g | Sugar: 1g | Protein: 2g

Note: The use of green parts of spring onions and careful choice of vegetables helps to keep this recipe FODMAP-friendly. Always ensure to adjust portion sizes based on your individual tolerance.

Preparation time: 15 minutes | Cooking time: 0 minutes | Makes: 4 servings

Ingredients:

- 4 ripe tomatoes, diced
- 1/2 cup green onions (green parts only), chopped
- 1/4 cup fresh cilantro, finely chopped
- 1 jalapeno pepper, seeds removed and finely chopped
- Juice of 1 lime
- Salt to taste

Instructions:

1. In a bowl, combine the diced tomatoes, chopped green onions, chopped cilantro, and finely chopped jalapeno pepper.
2. Add the juice of 1 lime and salt to taste. Stir until well mixed.
3. Cover and let it rest for at least 30 minutes to allow flavors to meld together.
4. Serve with low FODMAP tortilla chips or use as a topping on low FODMAP tacos.

Nutritional Values: Calories: 30 | Fat: 0g | Carbohydrates: 7g | Fiber: 2g | Sugar: 4g | Protein: 1g

Note: This recipe avoids garlic and onion, common in many salsa recipes but high in FODMAPs. The green parts of green onions are used as a low FODMAP alternative. Always adjust portion sizes according to individual tolerance levels.

DESSERTS RECIPES

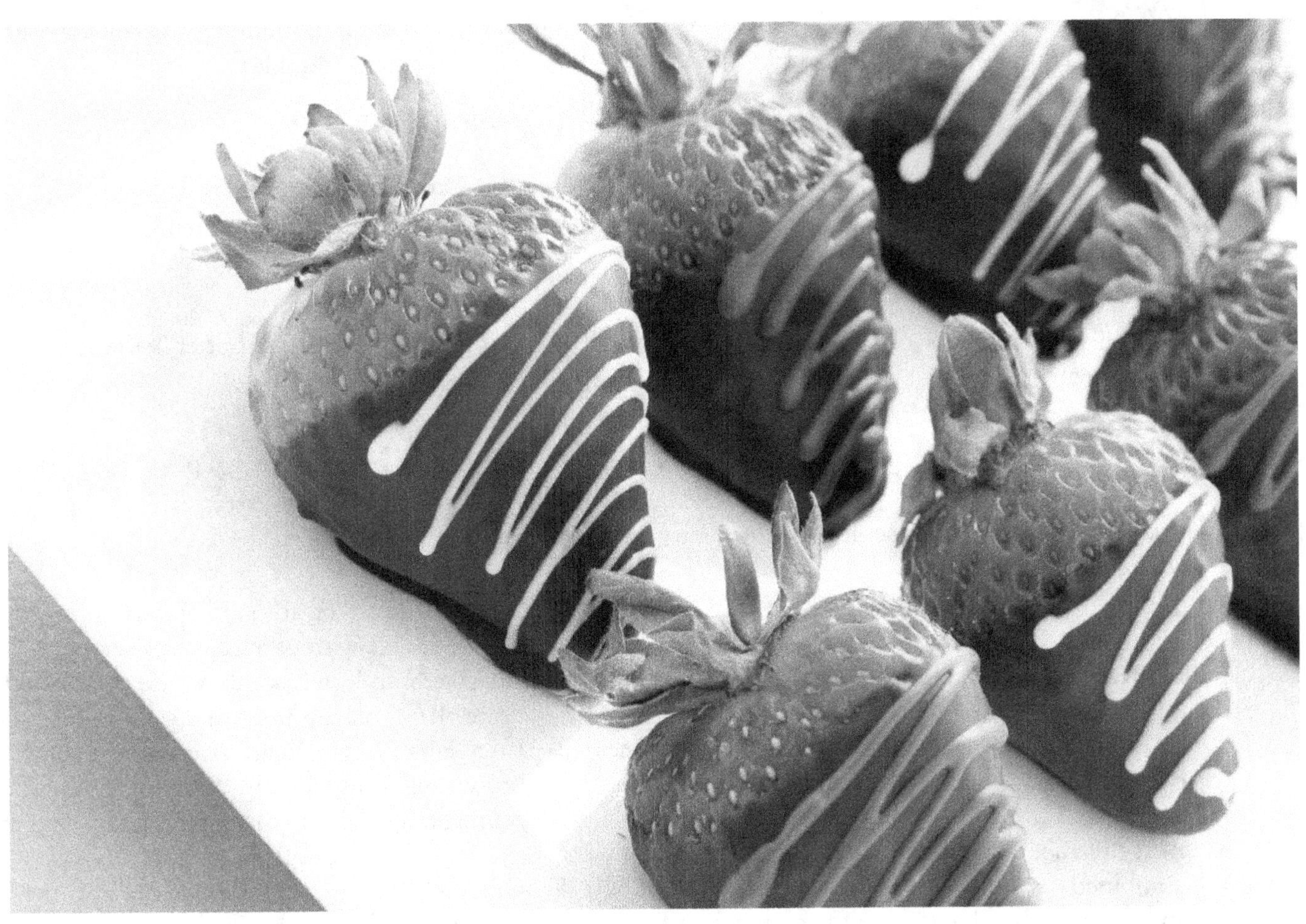

81. FODMAP-FRIENDLY CHOCOLATE CHIP COOKIES (V)

Preparation Time: 15 minutes | Cooking Time: 15 minutes | Yield: 20 cookies

Ingredients:

- 1 cup of gluten-free flour
- 1/2 cup of lactose-free butter, softened
- 3/4 cup of brown sugar
- 1/4 cup of caster sugar
- 1 large egg
- 1 tsp of pure vanilla extract
- 1/2 tsp of baking soda
- 1/4 tsp of salt
- 1 cup of dark chocolate chips (ensure dairy-free for vegan)

Directions:

1. Preheat your oven to 350°F (180°C) and line two baking trays with parchment paper.
2. In a large bowl, cream together the lactose-free butter, brown sugar, and caster sugar until light and fluffy.
3. Beat in the egg and vanilla extract until well combined.
4. In a separate bowl, combine the gluten-free flour, baking soda, and salt. Gradually add these dry ingredients to the butter mixture, beating well after each addition.
5. Stir in the chocolate chips.
6. Drop rounded tablespoons of the dough onto the prepared baking trays. Flatten slightly with the back of a spoon.
7. Bake for 10-15 minutes, or until golden brown. Allow the cookies to cool on the baking trays for 5 minutes before transferring them to wire racks to cool completely.

Nutritional Values (Per cookie): Calories: 125 | Protein: 1.6g | Carbs: 17.5g | Fat: 6.5g | Fiber: 0.9g | Sugar: 11.5g

82. LOW FODMAP MAPLE OATMEAL COOKIES

Preparation Time: 20 minutes | Cooking Time: 15 minutes | Yield: 24 cookies

Ingredients:

- 1 1/2 cups of gluten-free rolled oats
- 1 cup of gluten-free flour blend
- 1/2 teaspoon of baking soda
- 1/4 teaspoon of salt
- 1/2 cup of lactose-free butter, softened
- 3/4 cup of brown sugar
- 2 large eggs
- 1/4 cup of pure maple syrup
- 1 teaspoon of vanilla extract

Directions:

1. Preheat your oven to 350°F (180°C) and line two baking sheets with parchment paper.
2. In a medium bowl, combine the oats, gluten-free flour blend, baking soda, and salt.
3. In a large bowl, beat together the butter and brown sugar until creamy. Beat in the eggs, one at a time, then stir in the maple syrup and vanilla extract.
4. Gradually mix the dry ingredients into the butter mixture until well combined.
5. Drop rounded tablespoons of the dough onto the prepared baking sheets, spacing them about 2 inches apart.
6. Bake for 12-15 minutes, or until the edges are golden brown. Allow the cookies to cool on the baking sheets for 5 minutes before transferring them to wire racks to cool completely.

Nutritional Values (Per cookie): Calories: 120 | Protein: 2g | Carbs: 18g | Fat: 5g | Fiber: 1g | Sugar: 10g

Preparation Time: 20 minutes | Cooking Time: 40 minutes | Yield: 6 servings

Ingredients:

- 2 cups of chopped fresh strawberries
- 2 cups of chopped fresh rhubarb
- 1/2 cup of granulated sugar
- 2 tablespoons of cornstarch
- 1 cup of gluten-free rolled oats
- 1/2 cup of gluten-free flour blend
- 1/2 cup of packed brown sugar
- 1/2 teaspoon of ground cinnamon
- 1/3 cup of lactose-free butter, melted

Directions:

1. Preheat your oven to 350°F (180°C) and lightly grease a 9-inch square baking dish.
2. In a large bowl, combine the strawberries, rhubarb, granulated sugar, and cornstarch. Toss until the fruit is well coated, then pour into the prepared baking dish.
3. In another bowl, mix the oats, gluten-free flour blend, brown sugar, and cinnamon. Pour the melted butter over the top and stir until the mixture forms crumbles.
4. Sprinkle the crumble mixture evenly over the fruit in the baking dish.
5. Bake for 35-40 minutes, or until the crumble is golden brown and the fruit is bubbling. Allow to cool for a few minutes before serving.

Nutritional Values (Per serving): Calories: 300 | Protein: 3g | Carbs: 54g | Fat: 9g | Fiber: 3g | Sugar: 37g

Preparation Time: 20 minutes | Cooking Time: 25 minutes | Yield: 8 servings

Ingredients:

- 2 cups of gluten-free all-purpose flour
- 1/3 cup of granulated sugar
- 1 tablespoon of baking powder
- 1/2 teaspoon of baking soda
- 1/2 teaspoon of salt
- 1/2 cup of lactose-free butter, cold and cubed
- 2/3 cup of lactose-free milk
- 1 tablespoon of freshly grated lemon zest
- 1 cup of fresh blueberries
- 1 tablespoon of lemon juice
- 1 cup of confectioner's sugar

Directions:

1. Preheat your oven to 425°F (220°C). Line a baking sheet with parchment paper.
2. In a large bowl, combine the flour, sugar, baking powder, baking soda, and salt.
3. Cut the cold butter into the flour mixture using a pastry cutter or your fingers until the mixture resembles coarse crumbs.
4. Stir in the lactose-free milk and lemon zest until just combined. Gently fold in the blueberries.
5. Turn the dough out onto a lightly floured surface and knead it a few times to bring it together. Pat the dough into a 1-inch thick rectangle.
6. Cut the rectangle into 8 triangles and place them onto the prepared baking sheet.
7. Bake for 20-25 minutes, or until the scones are golden brown.
8. While the scones are baking, whisk together the lemon juice and confectioner's sugar to make a glaze.
9. Once the scones are cooled slightly, drizzle the glaze over the top.

Nutritional Values: Calories: 280 | Protein: 3g | Carbs: 45g | Fat: 10g | Fiber: 2g | Sugar: 20g

Preparation Time: 10 minutes | Freezing Time: 4 hours | Yield: 6 servings

Ingredients:

- 2 cups of fresh pineapple chunks
- 1 can (13.5 ounces) of coconut milk (Ensure that it does not contain any inulin or chicory root)
- 1/4 cup of maple syrup
- 1 teaspoon of pure vanilla extract
- Pinch of salt

Directions:

1. In a blender, combine the pineapple chunks, coconut milk, maple syrup, vanilla extract, and a pinch of salt.
2. Blend until smooth.
3. Pour the mixture into popsicle molds, leaving a little space at the top for them to expand.
4. Insert sticks into the molds and freeze for at least 4 hours, or until solid.
5. To remove the popsicles from the molds, run warm water on the outside of the molds for a few seconds, then gently pull the sticks.

Nutritional Values: Calories: 195 | Protein: 2g | Carbs: 18g | Fat: 14g | Fiber: 2g | Sugar: 14g

Note: Please note that while pineapple is considered low FODMAP, it contains naturally occurring sugars that could trigger symptoms in some people. Always listen to your body and modify recipes to suit your personal tolerance levels. If you are lactose intolerant, rest assured that coconut milk is a lactose-free ingredient.

Preparation Time: 20 minutes | Cooking Time: 25 minutes | Yield: 12 servings

Ingredients:

- 1 cup of almond meal (Almonds are low FODMAP in servings of 10 nuts or less. In this recipe, the almond meal is distributed among enough servings to stay within safe limits.)
- 1 cup of gluten-free flour blend
- 1 1/2 teaspoons of baking powder
- 1/2 teaspoon of baking soda
- 1/4 teaspoon of salt
- 3/4 cup of lactose-free milk
- 1/2 cup of pure maple syrup
- 1/4 cup of vegetable oil
- 2 large eggs
- 1 teaspoon of pure vanilla extract

Directions:

1. Preheat your oven to 350°F (180°C), and line a 12-cup muffin tin with paper liners.
2. In a large bowl, combine the almond meal, gluten-free flour blend, baking powder, baking soda, and salt.
3. In another bowl, whisk together the lactose-free milk, maple syrup, vegetable oil, eggs, and vanilla extract.
4. Gradually add the wet ingredients to the dry, stirring until just combined.
5. Divide the batter evenly among the prepared muffin cups.
6. Bake for 20-25 minutes, or until a toothpick inserted into the center of a muffin comes out clean.
7. Allow the muffins to cool in the tin for 5 minutes, then transfer them to a wire rack to cool completely.

Nutritional Values: Calories: 185 | Protein: 5g | Carbs: 21g | Fat: 10g | Fiber: 2g | Sugar: 10g

Preparation Time: 15 minutes | Cooking Time: 25 minutes | Yield: 24 cookies

Ingredients:

- 2 cups of gluten-free flour blend
- 1/4 teaspoon of salt
- 1 cup of unsalted butter, room temperature
- 1/2 cup of light brown sugar
- 1 teaspoon of pure vanilla extract

Directions:

1. Preheat your oven to 325°F (165°C) and line a baking sheet with parchment paper.
2. In a medium bowl, whisk together the gluten-free flour blend and salt.
3. In a large bowl, beat the butter until it's creamy and smooth. Add the brown sugar and continue to beat until it is fully incorporated. Beat in the vanilla extract.
4. Gradually add the flour mixture to the butter mixture, beating just until incorporated.
5. Flatten the dough into a disk shape, wrap in plastic wrap, and chill the dough for at least an hour or until firm.
6. On a lightly floured surface, roll out the dough to a thickness of 1/4 inch (0.5 cm). Using a cookie cutter, cut out cookies and place them onto the prepared baking sheet.
7. Bake for about 15-20 minutes or until cookies are browned around the edges. Remove from oven and cool on a wire rack.

Nutritional Values (Per cookie): Calories: 100 | Protein: 1g | Carbs: 10g | Fat: 6g | Fiber: 0g | Sugar: 4g

Preparation Time: 10 minutes | Cooking Time: 30 minutes | Yield: 4 servings

Ingredients:

- 4 ripe pears, any variety
- 4 teaspoons of pure maple syrup
- 1/2 teaspoon of ground cinnamon
- A pinch of salt
- 2 teaspoons of lactose-free butter or margarine

Directions:

1. Preheat your oven to 350°F (175°C) and line a baking sheet with parchment paper.
2. Cut the pears in half and remove the core. Place the pear halves on the baking sheet with the cut side up.
3. Drizzle each pear half with 1 teaspoon of maple syrup, sprinkle with a bit of cinnamon and a pinch of salt.
4. Put a small amount (about 1/2 teaspoon) of the lactose-free butter or margarine in the center of each pear.
5. Bake in the preheated oven for about 30 minutes or until the pears are tender. Serve warm.

Nutritional Values: Calories: 130 | Protein: 1g | Carbs: 32g | Fat: 2g | Fiber: 6g | Sugar: 22g

Preparation Time: 20 minutes | Cooking Time: 60 minutes | Chill Time: 4 hours | Yield: 12 servings

Ingredients:

- 2 cups of gluten-free graham crackers crumbs
- 1/2 cup of lactose-free butter, melted
- 3 cups of lactose-free cream cheese, at room temperature
- 1 cup of granulated sugar
- 3 large eggs
- 2 tablespoons of gluten-free cornstarch
- Zest and juice of 2 lemons
- 1 teaspoon of vanilla extract

Directions:

1. Preheat the oven to 325°F (165°C). Combine the graham cracker crumbs with the melted butter and press into the bottom of a 9-inch springform pan.
2. In a large bowl, beat the cream cheese until it is smooth. Gradually add the sugar, and then beat in the eggs one at a time.
3. Mix in the cornstarch, lemon zest, lemon juice, and vanilla extract. Pour this mixture over the crust in the springform pan.
4. Bake for 60 minutes, or until the cheesecake is set and the top is slightly browned. Let it cool on a wire rack for an hour, and then chill in the refrigerator for at least 4 hours before serving.

Nutritional Values: Calories: 370 | Protein: 6g | Carbs: 30g | Fat: 26g | Fiber: 1g | Sugar: 20g

Preparation Time: 15 minutes | Setting Time: 20 minutes | Yield: 16 strawberries

Ingredients:

- 16 fresh strawberries
- 1 cup of dairy-free dark chocolate chips

Directions:

1. Line a baking sheet with parchment paper.
2. Wash the strawberries and pat them dry. Make sure they are completely dry before you dip them into the chocolate.
3. Melt the chocolate chips in a microwave-safe bowl in 30-second increments, stirring each time until smooth.
4. Dip each strawberry into the melted chocolate, twirling it around to cover most of the strawberry.
5. Place each dipped strawberry onto the prepared baking sheet.
6. Once all strawberries are dipped, place the baking sheet in the refrigerator for 20 minutes, or until the chocolate has hardened.
7. Serve immediately, or store in an airtight container in the refrigerator until ready to serve.

Nutritional Values: Calories: 52 | Protein: 0.5g | Carbs: 6g | Fat: 3g | Fiber: 0.9g | Sugar: 4g

91. LOW FODMAP CITRUS PANNA COTTA (V)

Preparation Time: 10 minutes | Cooking Time: 10 minutes | Serves: 4

Ingredients:

- Zest and juice of 1 lemon
- Zest and juice of 1 orange
- 2 cups of lactose-free full-fat cream
- 1/4 cup of maple syrup
- 1 tablespoon of pure vanilla extract
- 2 1/4 teaspoons of unflavored gelatin
- Pinch of salt
- Fresh mint leaves, for garnish (optional)

Instructions:

1. In a small bowl, combine the orange and lemon juice. Sprinkle the gelatin over the juice and let it sit for about 5 minutes to soften.
2. Meanwhile, in a medium saucepan, combine the lactose-free cream, maple syrup, citrus zests, and a pinch of salt. Bring the mixture to a simmer over medium heat, stirring often.
3. Once simmering, remove the cream mixture from the heat. Add the softened gelatin and citrus juice to the cream, stirring until the gelatin is completely dissolved.
4. Pour the panna cotta mixture into four serving glasses or ramekins. Let them cool slightly at room temperature, then cover with plastic wrap and refrigerate until set, which should take at least 4 hours or overnight.
5. Before serving, garnish with fresh mint leaves, if desired.

Nutritional Values: 250 Calories | 22g Fat | 12g Carbohydrates | 3g Protein

92. FODMAP-FRIENDLY STRAWBERRY PARFAIT

Preparation Time: 10 minutes | No Cooking Time| Yield: 2 servings

Ingredients:

- 2 cups strawberries, sliced
- 1 cup lactose-free yogurt (ensure no high FODMAP ingredients added)
- 1 cup low FODMAP granola (without high FODMAP ingredients like cashews, pistachios, wheat, barley, and high FODMAP sweeteners)
- 1 teaspoon vanilla extract
- 1 tablespoon maple syrup

Directions:

1. In a bowl, mix the lactose-free yogurt with the vanilla extract and maple syrup.
2. Layer 1/4 of the yogurt mixture into the bottom of two glasses.
3. Follow with a layer of granola and then a layer of sliced strawberries.
4. Repeat the layers until the glasses are filled.
5. Top with a sprinkle of granola and a few strawberry slices.
6. Serve immediately and enjoy or refrigerate for up to 2 hours.

Nutritional Values: Calories: 320 | Protein: 12g | Carbs: 50g | Fat: 10g | Fiber: 5g | Sugar: 20g

Preparation Time: 5 minutes | No Cooking Time | Yield: 1 serving

Ingredients:

- 1 cup strawberries, frozen
- 1 cup lactose-free yogurt (ensure no high FODMAP ingredients added)
- 1 tablespoon chia seeds
- 1 tablespoon maple syrup

Directions:

1. In a blender, add the frozen strawberries, lactose-free yogurt, chia seeds, and maple syrup.
2. Blend until smooth and creamy. If the smoothie is too thick, add a bit of water or lactose-free milk to reach your desired consistency.
3. Pour into a glass, serve immediately, and enjoy!

Nutritional Values: Calories: 230 | Protein: 10g | Carbs: 35g | Fat: 5g | Fiber: 8g | Sugar: 20g

Preparation Time: 20 minutes | Cooking Time: 20 minutes | Yield: 12 cupcakes

Ingredients:

- 1 3/4 cups of gluten-free baking flour
- 1 cup of granulated sugar
- 1 teaspoon of baking powder
- 1/2 teaspoon of baking soda
- 1/2 teaspoon of salt
- 1 cup of almond milk
- 1/2 cup of vegetable oil
- 2 teaspoons of pure vanilla extract

For the Buttercream Frosting:

- 1/2 cup of dairy-free butter
- 2 cups of powdered sugar
- 2 teaspoons of pure vanilla extract
- 1-2 tablespoons of almond milk

Directions:

1. Preheat your oven to 350°F (175°C) and line a muffin tin with cupcake liners.
2. In a large bowl, mix the gluten-free flour, sugar, baking powder, baking soda, and salt.
3. In a separate bowl, whisk together the almond milk, vegetable oil, and vanilla extract.
4. Slowly add the wet ingredients into the dry ingredients, mixing until just combined.
5. Pour the batter into the lined muffin tin, filling each about 3/4 full.
6. Bake for about 20 minutes, or until a toothpick inserted into the center comes out clean. Let the cupcakes cool completely before frosting.

For the Buttercream Frosting:

1. Beat the dairy-free butter until soft and creamy. Gradually add in the powdered sugar, vanilla extract, and almond milk as needed, until you reach your desired consistency.
2. Once the cupcakes are cooled, frost them with the buttercream frosting.

Nutritional Values (Per cupcake): Calories: 250 | Protein: 2g | Carbs: 35g | Fat: 12g | Fiber: 1g | Sugar: 22g

95. CHIA SEED PUDDING WITH BLUEBERRIES (VG)

Preparation Time: 10 minutes | Refrigeration Time: 4 hours (or overnight) | Yield: 4 servings

Ingredients:

- 1/2 cup of chia seeds
- 2 cups of almond milk, unsweetened
- 1 tablespoon of pure maple syrup
- 1 teaspoon of pure vanilla extract
- 1 cup of fresh blueberries

Directions:

1. In a bowl, mix the chia seeds, almond milk, maple syrup, and vanilla extract.
2. Stir well to ensure there are no clumps, and the chia seeds are evenly distributed.
3. Cover the bowl and place it in the refrigerator for at least 4 hours, or overnight, until the chia seeds have absorbed the liquid and formed a pudding-like texture.
4. When ready to serve, give the chia seed pudding a good stir. If it is too thick, add a bit more almond milk.
5. Divide the chia seed pudding into four servings, and top each with a quarter of the fresh blueberries.

Nutritional Values: Calories: 175 | Protein: 5g | Carbs: 20g | Fat: 9g | Fiber: 9g | Sugar: 7g

96. LOW FODMAP BLUEBERRY PIE

Preparation Time: 30 minutes | Baking Time: 50 minutes | Yield: 8 servings

Ingredients:

- 1 1/2 cups of gluten-free flour
- 1/2 teaspoon of salt
- 1/2 cup of cold unsalted butter, cubed
- 3-4 tablespoons of ice water
- 4 cups of fresh blueberries
- 1/2 cup of white sugar
- 2 tablespoons of cornstarch
- 1 teaspoon of cinnamon
- 1 tablespoon of lemon juice
- 1 egg, beaten (for egg wash)

Directions:

1. Combine the gluten-free flour and salt in a bowl. Cut in the cold butter using a pastry blender or your fingers until the mixture resembles coarse crumbs. Add ice water, one tablespoon at a time, until the dough comes together.
2. Divide the dough into two equal parts, shape them into disks, and wrap them in plastic wrap. Refrigerate for at least 30 minutes.
3. Preheat your oven to 375°F (190°C).
4. Roll out one of the dough disks on a lightly floured surface to fit your pie dish. Transfer the dough into the dish and trim the excess.
5. In a separate bowl, combine the blueberries, sugar, cornstarch, cinnamon, and lemon juice. Pour this mixture into the pie crust.
6. Roll out the second disk of dough and place it over the blueberries. Trim, fold, and crimp the edges, then cut small slits in the top crust to vent. Brush the crust with the beaten egg.
7. Bake the pie in the preheated oven for about 50 minutes, or until the crust is golden and the filling is bubbling. Allow the pie to cool before serving.

Nutritional Values: Calories: 285 | Protein: 3g | Carbs: 40g | Fat: 13g | Fiber: 3g | Sugar: 18g

97. FODMAP-FRIENDLY CHOCOLATE MOUSSE

Preparation Time: 15 minutes | Chilling Time: 2 hours | Yield: 4 servings

Ingredients:

- 200g dark chocolate (ensure it is lactose-free and low FODMAP)
- 2 tablespoons of granulated sugar
- 3 large eggs, separated
- A pinch of salt
- 1/2 teaspoon of vanilla extract
- Fresh strawberries for garnish (ensure to limit serving size to avoid FODMAP overload)

Directions:

1. Melt the chocolate slowly in a heatproof bowl over simmering water, stirring occasionally. Once melted, remove from heat, and let cool slightly.
2. Meanwhile, in a large bowl, beat the egg yolks, sugar, and vanilla extract until creamy and light.
3. Gradually mix the melted chocolate into the egg yolk mixture until well combined.
4. In another bowl, whisk the egg whites and salt until soft peaks form.
5. Gently fold the egg whites into the chocolate mixture, making sure it is well incorporated but also trying to keep as much air in the mixture as possible.
6. Divide the mousse among 4 individual serving dishes, cover, and refrigerate for at least 2 hours or until set.
7. Before serving, garnish with fresh strawberries, but remember to stick to a low FODMAP serving size of no more than 140g per serving to avoid triggering symptoms.

Nutritional Values: Calories: 315 | Protein: 7g | Carbs: 22g | Fat: 23g | Fiber: 3g | Sugar: 16g

98. LOW FODMAP RASPBERRY COCONUT MACAROONS (VG)

Preparation Time: 15 minutes | Cooking Time: 20 minutes | Serves: 20

Ingredients:

- 2 cups of shredded unsweetened coconut
- 1/2 cup of fresh blueberries
- 1/4 cup of pure maple syrup
- 2 tablespoons of coconut flour
- 2 tablespoons of chia seeds
- 1 teaspoon of pure vanilla extract
- Pinch of salt

Instructions:

1. Preheat your oven to 350°F (175°C) and line a baking sheet with parchment paper.
2. In a large bowl, combine the shredded coconut, blueberries, maple syrup, coconut flour, chia seeds, vanilla extract, and a pinch of salt. Stir until all the ingredients are well mixed.
3. Scoop tablespoon-sized mounds of the coconut mixture onto the prepared baking sheet, pressing each mound together firmly.
4. Bake in the preheated oven for 20 minutes, or until the edges of the macaroons are golden brown.
5. Allow the macaroons to cool on the baking sheet for 10 minutes, then transfer to a wire rack to cool completely before serving.

Nutritional Values: 80 Calories | 6g Fat | 6g Carbohydrates | 1g Protein

Note: Since raspberries are not permitted in a low FODMAP diet, I have replaced them with blueberries which are considered low FODMAP in lesser amounts.

99. FODMAP-friendly Raspberry Sorbet (VG)

Preparation Time: 10 minutes | Freezing Time: 4 hours | Yield: 4 servings

Ingredients:

- 4 cups of strawberries
- 1/4 cup of maple syrup
- 2 tablespoons of fresh lemon juice
- A pinch of salt

Directions:

1. Rinse and hull the strawberries.
2. In a blender, add strawberries, maple syrup, lemon juice, and a pinch of salt. Blend until smooth.
3. Pour the mixture into a shallow dish and cover it with plastic wrap.
4. Freeze for about 1 hour, then stir with a fork to break up any ice crystals starting to form.
5. Continue to freeze, stirring once every hour, until the sorbet is frozen, about 3 to 4 hours.
6. Before serving, let it stand at room temperature until slightly softened.
7. Serve the sorbet in dessert dishes, garnishing with a few additional strawberries if desired.

Nutritional Values: Calories: 100 | Protein: 1g | Carbs: 25g | Fat: 0g | Fiber: 2g | Sugar: 21g

100. Low FODMAP Mint Chocolate Chip Ice Cream

Preparation Time: 15 minutes | Freezing Time: 6 hours | Yield: 8 servings

Ingredients:

- 2 cans (400 ml each) full-fat coconut milk
- 1/2 cup maple syrup
- 2 tsp pure peppermint extract
- 1/2 cup dark chocolate chips (ensure they are dairy-free if you are lactose intolerant)

Directions:

1. In a blender, combine the coconut milk, maple syrup, and peppermint extract. Blend until the mixture is smooth and well combined.
2. Pour the mixture into an ice cream maker and churn according to the manufacturer's instructions.
3. When the mixture has thickened and looks like soft serve, add in the chocolate chips, and churn a few more minutes to incorporate.
4. Transfer the ice cream to a lidded container. Cover and freeze until firm, at least 4-6 hours or overnight.
5. Let it sit at room temperature for a few minutes before scooping and serving.

Nutritional Values: Calories: 280 | Protein: 2g | Carbs: 23g | Fat: 20g | Fiber: 0g | Sugar: 18g

CONCLUSION

Living with Irritable Bowel Syndrome (IBS) is a complex journey, but it's also a path to improved health, better quality of life, and self-discovery. The low-FODMAP diet is a crucial tool for managing IBS symptoms. Despite its challenges, this diet can provide substantial relief and significantly improve your quality of life.

Navigating the intricacies of this diet demands resilience, patience, and determination. Embracing the journey involves acknowledging the challenges, recognizing your strengths, and maintaining a forward-looking perspective. Living with IBS can be tricky dealing with unpredictable symptoms, adjusting to dietary changes, and facing their impact on daily life. Recognizing these difficulties and understanding that having tough days and setbacks is okay is essential. These challenges can serve as steppingstones toward progress and resilience.

Adopting a self-compassionate approach is critical to making this journey more manageable. Self-compassion means being kind and understanding towards yourself in times of pain or failure rather than being overly critical. This perspective allows for patience when changes don't happen immediately or when setbacks occur, fostering a positive mindset.

In this journey, arming yourself with accurate knowledge about IBS and the Low-FODMAP diet is not just information, it's power. Understanding your condition, its potential triggers, how it affects your body, and how the diet operates empowers you to take charge of your health. Furthermore, staying abreast of the latest research can provide you with new tools for better symptom management, thus nurturing hope for a healthier future.

You don't have to navigate this journey alone - building a support system is not just helpful; it's crucial in effectively managing IBS. This can include a range of people, from medical professionals, dietitians, and mental health experts to family, friends, and support groups. A strong support system can provide a sense of community, emotional support, practical help, and valuable advice, making the journey less daunting and more manageable.

Maintaining a positive outlook and staying motivated are equally essential. Focusing on your progress rather than aiming for perfection, cultivating a positive mindset, setting achievable goals, and seeking support when needed can foster resilience, motivate you to continue the journey, and lead to better health.

While it is essential to appreciate the progress made and stay in the present, it is also important to maintain a forward-looking perspective. Anticipate future advancements in IBS research, remain flexible to adapt to recent changes, and continue prioritizing self-care.

Appreciating the journey you have embarked on is vital. It takes great bravery and persistence to educate yourself about IBS and make changes to your diet. Every step you take is a testament to your strength. Your journey with IBS is a path of self-discovery. Embrace it, learn from it, and remember that every step you take brings you closer to better health and an improved quality of life.

In conclusion, managing IBS and following the low-FODMAP diet is challenging but rewarding. It is a path towards better health, self-understanding, and improved quality of life. While this journey demands patience, resilience, and strength, it offers hope and empowerment. You are not alone on this journey. With your learned strategies, you can navigate your way, manage your symptoms, and lead a vibrant, fulfilling life. Keep going, believe in yourself, and know that every step forward is not just a step, it's a leap towards better health and a brighter future.

APPENDIX

28-DAY LOW FODMAP MEAL PLAN

<table>
<tr><td colspan="2">DAY 1:</td><td colspan="2">DAY 4:</td></tr>
<tr><td>Breakfast:</td><td>Quick and Easy Banana Pancakes (V)</td><td>Breakfast:</td><td>Egg and Cheddar Breakfast Wrap</td></tr>
<tr><td>Snack/Dessert:</td><td>Chia Seed and Blueberry Energy Balls (VG)</td><td>Snack/Dessert:</td><td>Maple Cinnamon Baked Pears</td></tr>
<tr><td>Lunch:</td><td>Baked Lemon Chicken with Thyme</td><td>Lunch:</td><td>Quinoa Salad with Grilled Veggies (V)</td></tr>
<tr><td>Snack/Dessert:</td><td>Low FODMAP Citrus Panna Cotta (V)</td><td>Snack/Dessert:</td><td>Low FODMAP Almond Muffins</td></tr>
<tr><td>Dinner:</td><td>Grilled Lemon Dill Salmon</td><td>Dinner:</td><td>Garlic Infused Olive Oil Shrimp Scampi</td></tr>
</table>

<table>
<tr><td colspan="2">DAY 2:</td><td colspan="2">DAY 5:</td></tr>
<tr><td>Breakfast:</td><td>Overnight Chia Pudding with Berries (VG)</td><td>Breakfast:</td><td>Buckwheat Banana Muffins (V)</td></tr>
<tr><td>Snack/Dessert:</td><td>Baked Feta with Cherry Tomatoes (V)</td><td>Snack/Dessert:</td><td>FODMAP-friendly Strawberry Parfait</td></tr>
<tr><td>Lunch:</td><td>Grilled Salmon with Dill Sauce</td><td>Lunch:</td><td>Tuna and Rice Salad with Lemon Vinaigrette</td></tr>
<tr><td>Snack/Dessert:</td><td>Low FODMAP Raspberry Coconut Macaroons (VG)</td><td>Snack/Dessert:</td><td>Chocolate Dipped Strawberries (VG)</td></tr>
<tr><td>Dinner:</td><td>Thai Basil Beef Stir Fry</td><td>Dinner:</td><td>Grilled Steak with Chimichurri Sauce</td></tr>
</table>

<table>
<tr><td colspan="2">DAY 3:</td><td colspan="2">DAY 6:</td></tr>
<tr><td>Breakfast:</td><td>Quinoa Breakfast Porridge (V)</td><td>Breakfast:</td><td>Fruit & Nut Granola with Lactose-free Yogurt (V)</td></tr>
<tr><td>Snack/Dessert:</td><td>Pineapple Coconut Popsicles (VG)</td><td>Snack/Dessert:</td><td>Low FODMAP Blueberry Pie</td></tr>
<tr><td>Lunch:</td><td>Low-FODMAP Chicken Stir-Fry</td><td>Lunch:</td><td>Gluten-free Pasta with Garlic Infused Olive Oil and Chili (V)</td></tr>
<tr><td>Snack/Dessert:</td><td>FODMAP-friendly Lemon Poppy Seed Muffins</td><td>Snack/Dessert:</td><td>FODMAP-friendly Lemon Cheesecake</td></tr>
<tr><td>Dinner:</td><td>Teriyaki Chicken Skewers with Pineapple Salsa</td><td>Dinner:</td><td>Oven-Baked Rosemary Chicken Thighs</td></tr>
</table>

DAY 7:

Breakfast:	Healthy Spinach and Tomato Omelette
Snack/Dessert:	Simple Vanilla Cupcakes with Buttercream Frosting (V)
Lunch:	Low-FODMAP Beef Tacos
Snack/Dessert:	Low FODMAP Mint Chocolate Chip Ice Cream
Dinner:	Rainbow Quinoa Salad with Lemon Vinaigrette (VG)

DAY 8:

Breakfast:	Buckwheat Banana Muffins (V)
Snack/Dessert:	Low FODMAP Citrus Panna Cotta (V)
Lunch:	Low-FODMAP Beef Tacos
Snack/Dessert:	Pineapple Coconut Popsicles (VG)
Dinner:	Maple Glazed Roast Pork with Carrots

DAY 9:

Breakfast:	Fruit & Nut Granola with Lactose-free Yogurt (V)
Snack/Dessert:	Low FODMAP Raspberry Coconut Macaroons (VG)
Lunch:	Zucchini Noodles with Shrimp
Snack/Dessert:	Low FODMAP Almond Muffins
Dinner:	Baked Cod with Tomato and Basil

DAY 10:

Breakfast:	Healthy Spinach and Tomato Omelette
Snack/Dessert:	Low FODMAP Mint Chocolate Chip Ice Cream
Lunch:	Greek Salad with Grilled Chicken
Snack/Dessert:	Chia Seed and Blueberry Energy Balls (VG)
Dinner:	Quick Chicken and Vegetable Stir-Fry

DAY 11:

Breakfast:	Gluten-Free Waffles with Maple Syrup (V)
Snack/Dessert:	FODMAP-friendly Lemon Cheesecake
Lunch:	Egg Salad Lettuce Wraps (V)
Snack/Dessert:	FODMAP-friendly Lemon Poppy Seed Muffins
Dinner:	Grilled Steak with Chimichurri Sauce

DAY 12:

Breakfast:	Stuffed Bell Peppers with Scrambled Eggs
Snack/Dessert:	FODMAP-friendly Strawberry Parfait
Lunch:	Baked Cod with Lemon and Parsley
Snack/Dessert:	FODMAP-friendly Chocolate Mousse
Dinner:	Oven-Baked Rosemary Chicken Thighs

DAY 13:

Breakfast:	Buckwheat and Blueberry Breakfast Bowl (VG)
Snack/Dessert:	Pineapple Coconut Popsicles (VG)
Lunch:	Grilled Steak with Sautéed Green Beans
Snack/Dessert:	Low FODMAP Citrus Panna Cotta (V)
Dinner:	Beef and Red Pepper Stuffed Bell Peppers

DAY 14:

Breakfast:	Peanut Butter and Banana Smoothie (VG)
Snack/Dessert:	Low FODMAP Raspberry Coconut Macaroons (VG)
Lunch:	Easy Shrimp Fried Rice
Snack/Dessert:	Low FODMAP Almond Muffins
Dinner:	Roast Turkey Breast with Herbs and Lemon

DAY 15:

Breakfast:	FODMAP-friendly Breakfast Burrito
Snack/Dessert:	Chocolate Dipped Strawberries (VG)
Lunch:	Quinoa and Tofu Stuffed Peppers (VG)
Snack/Dessert:	Low FODMAP Mint Chocolate Chip Ice Cream
Dinner:	Shrimp and Pineapple Fried Rice

DAY 16:

Breakfast:	Oatmeal with Cinnamon and Grated Apple (VG)
Snack/Dessert:	Low FODMAP Citrus Panna Cotta (V)
Lunch:	Grilled Tuna Steaks with Olive Tapenade
Snack/Dessert:	FODMAP-friendly Lemon Cheesecake
Dinner:	Stir-Fried Tofu with Bell Peppers and Broccoli (VG)

DAY 17:

Breakfast:	Strawberry and Chia Seed Jam on Gluten-Free Toast (V)
Snack/Dessert:	Low FODMAP Raspberry Coconut Macaroons (VG)
Lunch:	Turkey and Swiss Lettuce Wraps
Snack/Dessert:	Brown Sugar Shortbread (V)
Dinner:	Baked Cod with Tomato and Basil

DAY 18:

Breakfast:	Bacon and Egg Breakfast Muffins
Snack/Dessert:	FODMAP-friendly Chocolate Mousse
Lunch:	Butternut Squash Soup (V)
Snack/Dessert:	Simple Vanilla Cupcakes with Buttercream Frosting (V)
Dinner:	Eggplant and Zucchini Ratatouille (VG)

DAY 19:

Breakfast:	Almond Milk Overnight Oats with Raspberries (VG)
Snack/Dessert:	Low FODMAP Maple Oatmeal Cookies
Lunch:	Sesame Ginger Stir-Fry with Tofu (VG)
Snack/Dessert:	Pineapple Coconut Popsicles (VG)
Dinner:	Thai Basil Beef Stir Fry

DAY 20:

Breakfast:	Sautéed Tomatoes and Spinach on Sourdough Toast (V)
Snack/Dessert:	Low FODMAP Blueberry Pie
Lunch:	Grilled Halibut with Lemon Herb Sauce
Snack/Dessert:	Chia Seed and Blueberry Energy Balls (VG)
Dinner:	Maple Glazed Roast Pork with Carrots

DAY 21:

Breakfast:	Quinoa and Zucchini Fritters (VG)
Snack/Dessert:	Strawberry Rhubarb Crumble (V)
Lunch:	Grilled Salmon with Dill Sauce
Snack/Dessert:	FODMAP-friendly Lemon Poppy Seed Muffins
Dinner:	Garlic Infused Olive Oil Shrimp Scampi

DAY 22:

Breakfast:	FODMAP-friendly Breakfast Burrito
Snack/Dessert:	FODMAP-friendly Raspberry Sorbet (VG)
Lunch:	Grilled Steak with Sautéed Green Beans
Snack/Dessert:	FODMAP-friendly Chocolate Chip Cookies (V)
Dinner:	Thai Basil Beef Stir Fry

DAY 23:

Breakfast:	Quinoa Breakfast Porridge (V)
Snack/Dessert:	Strawberry Rhubarb Crumble (V)
Lunch:	Easy Shrimp Fried Rice
Snack/Dessert:	Low FODMAP Citrus Panna Cotta (V)
Dinner:	Zucchini Noodles with Lemon Garlic Shrimp

DAY 24:

Breakfast:	Quick and Easy Banana Pancakes (V)
Snack/Dessert:	Pineapple Coconut Popsicles (VG)
Lunch:	Baked Lemon Chicken with Thyme
Snack/Dessert:	Low FODMAP Raspberry Coconut Macaroons (VG)
Dinner:	Rainbow Quinoa Salad with Lemon Vinaigrette (VG)

DAY 25:

Breakfast:	Stuffed Bell Peppers with Scrambled Eggs
Snack/Dessert:	Low FODMAP Blueberry Pie
Lunch:	Greek Salad with Grilled Chicken
Snack/Dessert:	FODMAP-friendly Lemon Cheesecake
Dinner:	Oven-Baked Lemon Thyme Salmon (V)

DAY 26:

Breakfast:	Gluten-Free Waffles with Maple Syrup (V)
Snack/Dessert:	Chocolate Dipped Strawberries (VG)
Lunch:	Quinoa Salad with Grilled Veggies (V)
Snack/Dessert:	Brown Sugar Shortbread (V)
Dinner:	Shrimp and Pineapple Fried Rice

DAY 27:

Breakfast:	Overnight Chia Pudding with Berries (VG)
Snack/Dessert:	FODMAP-friendly Chocolate Mousse
Lunch:	Tuna and Rice Salad with Lemon Vinaigrette
Snack/Dessert:	Low FODMAP Mint Chocolate Chip Ice Cream
Dinner:	Quick Chicken and Vegetable Stir-Fry

DAY 28:

Breakfast:	Almond Milk Overnight Oats with Raspberries (VG)
Snack/Dessert:	Low FODMAP Maple Oatmeal Cookies
Lunch:	Zucchini Noodles with Shrimp
Snack/Dessert:	Simple Vanilla Cupcakes with Buttercream Frosting (V)
Dinner:	Spaghetti Squash with Tomato Basil Sauce (V)

DAY 1:

Breakfast:	Quick and Easy Banana Pancakes (V)
Snack/Dessert:	Strawberry and Banana Smoothie Bowl (VG)
Lunch:	Sesame Ginger Stir-Fry with Tofu (VG)
Snack/Dessert:	Chia Seed and Blueberry Energy Balls (VG)
Dinner:	Spaghetti Squash with Tomato Basil Sauce (V)

DAY 2:

Breakfast:	Low-FODMAP Friendly Smoothie Bowl (V)
Snack/Dessert:	Oven-Baked Zucchini Chips with Dill Dip (V)
Lunch:	Quinoa Salad with Grilled Veggies (V)
Snack/Dessert:	Smoky Quinoa-Stuffed Mini Bell Peppers (VG)
Dinner:	Roasted Acorn Squash with Quinoa and Kale Stuffing (VG)

DAY 3:

Breakfast:	Buckwheat Banana Muffins (V)
Snack/Dessert:	Baked Feta with Cherry Tomatoes (V)
Lunch:	Egg Salad Lettuce Wraps (V)
Snack/Dessert:	Quick and Easy Carrot and Cucumber Sticks with Homemade Hummus (V)
Dinner:	Stir-Fried Tofu with Bell Peppers and Broccoli (VG)

DAY 4:

Breakfast:	Fruit & Nut Granola with Lactose-free Yogurt (V)
Snack/Dessert:	Smashed Avocado on Gluten-Free Toast (V)
Lunch:	Gluten-free Pasta with Garlic Infused Olive Oil and Chili (V)
Snack/Dessert:	Chia Seed and Blueberry Energy Balls (VG)
Dinner:	Oven-Baked Lemon Thyme Salmon (V)

DAY 5:

Breakfast:	Overnight Chia Pudding with Berries (VG)
Snack/Dessert:	Strawberry and Banana Smoothie Bowl (VG)
Lunch:	Quinoa and Tofu Stuffed Peppers (VG)
Snack/Dessert:	Oven-Baked Zucchini Chips with Dill Dip (V)
Dinner:	Eggplant and Zucchini Ratatouille (VG)

DAY 6:

Breakfast:	Almond Milk Overnight Oats with Raspberries (VG)
Snack/Dessert:	Smoky Quinoa-Stuffed Mini Bell Peppers (VG)
Lunch:	Butternut Squash Soup (V)
Snack/Dessert:	Quick and Easy Carrot and Cucumber Sticks with Homemade Hummus (V)
Dinner:	Rainbow Quinoa Salad with Lemon Vinaigrette (VG)

DAY 7:

Breakfast:	Gluten-Free Waffles with Maple Syrup (V)
Snack/Dessert:	Baked Feta with Cherry Tomatoes (V)
Lunch:	Quinoa Salad with Grilled Veggies (V)
Snack/Dessert:	Smashed Avocado on Gluten-Free Toast (V)
Dinner:	Spaghetti Squash with Tomato Basil Sauce (V)

DAY 8:

Breakfast:	Quinoa Breakfast Porridge (V)
Snack/Dessert:	Strawberry and Banana Smoothie Bowl (VG)
Lunch:	Egg Salad Lettuce Wraps (V)
Snack/Dessert:	Chia Seed and Blueberry Energy Balls (VG)
Dinner:	Stir-Fried Tofu with Bell Peppers and Broccoli (VG)

DAY 9:

Breakfast:	Quick and Easy Banana Pancakes (V)
Snack/Dessert:	Oven-Baked Zucchini Chips with Dill Dip (V)
Lunch:	Gluten-free Pasta with Garlic Infused Olive Oil and Chili (V)
Snack/Dessert:	Smoky Quinoa-Stuffed Mini Bell Peppers (VG)
Dinner:	Oven-Baked Lemon Thyme Salmon (V)

DAY 10:

Breakfast:	Overnight Chia Pudding with Berries (VG)
Snack/Dessert:	Baked Feta with Cherry Tomatoes (V)
Lunch:	Quinoa and Tofu Stuffed Peppers (VG)
Snack/Dessert:	Quick and Easy Carrot and Cucumber Sticks with Homemade Hummus (V)
Dinner:	Butternut Squash and Chicken Curry (V)

DAY 11:

Breakfast:	Buckwheat Banana Muffins (V)
Snack/Dessert:	Smashed Avocado on Gluten-Free Toast (V)
Lunch:	Quinoa Salad with Grilled Veggies (V)
Snack/Dessert:	Chia Seed and Blueberry Energy Balls (VG)
Dinner:	Rainbow Quinoa Salad with Lemon Vinaigrette (VG)

DAY 12:

Breakfast:	Fruit & Nut Granola with Lactose-free Yogurt (V)
Snack/Dessert:	Strawberry and Banana Smoothie Bowl (VG)
Lunch:	Sesame Ginger Stir-Fry with Tofu (VG)
Snack/Dessert:	Oven-Baked Zucchini Chips with Dill Dip (V)
Dinner:	Eggplant and Zucchini Ratatouille (VG)

DAY 13:

Breakfast:	Almond Milk Overnight Oats with Raspberries (VG)
Snack/Dessert:	Smoky Quinoa-Stuffed Mini Bell Peppers (VG)
Lunch:	Butternut Squash Soup (V)
Snack/Dessert:	Quick and Easy Carrot and Cucumber Sticks with Homemade Hummus (V)
Dinner:	Spaghetti Squash with Tomato Basil Sauce (V)

DAY 14:

Breakfast:	Gluten-Free Waffles with Maple Syrup (V)
Snack/Dessert:	Baked Feta with Cherry Tomatoes (V)
Lunch:	Egg Salad Lettuce Wraps (V)
Snack/Dessert:	Smashed Avocado on Gluten-Free Toast (V)
Dinner:	Stir-Fried Tofu with Bell Peppers and Broccoli (VG)

DAY 15:

Breakfast:	Low-FODMAP Friendly Smoothie Bowl (V)
Snack/Dessert:	Oven-Baked Zucchini Chips with Dill Dip (V)
Lunch:	Quinoa Salad with Grilled Veggies (V)
Snack/Dessert:	Smoky Quinoa-Stuffed Mini Bell Peppers (VG)
Dinner:	Roasted Acorn Squash with Quinoa and Kale Stuffing (VG)

DAY 16:

Breakfast:	Quick and Easy Banana Pancakes (V)
Snack/Dessert:	Strawberry and Banana Smoothie Bowl (VG)
Lunch:	Sesame Ginger Stir-Fry with Tofu (VG)
Snack/Dessert:	Chia Seed and Blueberry Energy Balls (VG)
Dinner:	Spaghetti Squash with Tomato Basil Sauce (V)

DAY 17:

Breakfast:	Fruit & Nut Granola with Lactose-free Yogurt (V)
Snack/Dessert:	Smashed Avocado on Gluten-Free Toast (V)
Lunch:	Gluten-free Pasta with Garlic Infused Olive Oil and Chili (V)
Snack/Dessert:	Chia Seed and Blueberry Energy Balls (VG)
Dinner:	Oven-Baked Lemon Thyme Salmon (V)

DAY 18:

Breakfast:	Buckwheat Banana Muffins (V)
Snack/Dessert:	Baked Feta with Cherry Tomatoes (V)
Lunch:	Egg Salad Lettuce Wraps (V)
Snack/Dessert:	Quick and Easy Carrot and Cucumber Sticks with Homemade Hummus (V)
Dinner:	Stir-Fried Tofu with Bell Peppers and Broccoli (VG)

DAY 19:

Breakfast:	Almond Milk Overnight Oats with Raspberries (VG)
Snack/Dessert:	Smoky Quinoa-Stuffed Mini Bell Peppers (VG)
Lunch:	Butternut Squash Soup (V)
Snack/Dessert:	Quick and Easy Carrot and Cucumber Sticks with Homemade Hummus (V)
Dinner:	Rainbow Quinoa Salad with Lemon Vinaigrette (VG)

DAY 20:

Breakfast:	Overnight Chia Pudding with Berries (VG)
Snack/Dessert:	Strawberry and Banana Smoothie Bowl (VG)
Lunch:	Quinoa and Tofu Stuffed Peppers (VG)
Snack/Dessert:	Oven-Baked Zucchini Chips with Dill Dip (V)
Dinner:	Eggplant and Zucchini Ratatouille (VG)

DAY 21:

Breakfast:	Gluten-Free Waffles with Maple Syrup (V)
Snack/Dessert:	Baked Feta with Cherry Tomatoes (V)
Lunch:	Quinoa Salad with Grilled Veggies (V)
Snack/Dessert:	Smashed Avocado on Gluten-Free Toast (V)
Dinner:	Spaghetti Squash with Tomato Basil Sauce (V)

DAY 22:

Breakfast:	Fruit & Nut Granola with Lactose-free Yogurt (V)
Snack/Dessert:	Strawberry and Banana Smoothie Bowl (VG)
Lunch:	Sesame Ginger Stir-Fry with Tofu (VG)
Snack/Dessert:	Oven-Baked Zucchini Chips with Dill Dip (V)
Dinner:	Eggplant and Zucchini Ratatouille (VG)

DAY 23:

Breakfast:	Buckwheat Banana Muffins (V)
Snack/Dessert:	Smashed Avocado on Gluten-Free Toast (V)
Lunch:	Quinoa Salad with Grilled Veggies (V)
Snack/Dessert:	Chia Seed and Blueberry Energy Balls (VG)
Dinner:	Rainbow Quinoa Salad with Lemon Vinaigrette (VG)

DAY 24:

Breakfast:	Gluten-Free Waffles with Maple Syrup (V)
Snack/Dessert:	Baked Feta with Cherry Tomatoes (V)
Lunch:	Egg Salad Lettuce Wraps (V)
Snack/Dessert:	Smashed Avocado on Gluten-Free Toast (V)
Dinner:	Stir-Fried Tofu with Bell Peppers and Broccoli (VG)

DAY 25:

Breakfast:	Quick and Easy Banana Pancakes (V)
Snack/Dessert:	Oven-Baked Zucchini Chips with Dill Dip (V)
Lunch:	Gluten-free Pasta with Garlic Infused Olive Oil and Chili (V)
Snack/Dessert:	Smoky Quinoa-Stuffed Mini Bell Peppers (VG)
Dinner:	Oven-Baked Lemon Thyme Salmon (V)

DAY 26:

Breakfast:	Quinoa Breakfast Porridge (V)
Snack/Dessert:	Strawberry and Banana Smoothie Bowl (VG)
Lunch:	Egg Salad Lettuce Wraps (V)
Snack/Dessert:	Chia Seed and Blueberry Energy Balls (VG)
Dinner:	Stir-Fried Tofu with Bell Peppers and Broccoli (VG)

DAY 27:

Breakfast:	Almond Milk Overnight Oats with Raspberries (VG)
Snack/Dessert:	Smoky Quinoa-Stuffed Mini Bell Peppers (VG)
Lunch:	Butternut Squash Soup (V)
Snack/Dessert:	Quick and Easy Carrot and Cucumber Sticks with Homemade Hummus (V)
Dinner:	Spaghetti Squash with Tomato Basil Sauce (V)

DAY 28:

Breakfast:	Overnight Chia Pudding with Berries (VG)
Snack/Dessert:	Baked Feta with Cherry Tomatoes (V)
Lunch:	Quinoa and Tofu Stuffed Peppers (VG)
Snack/Dessert:	Quick and Easy Carrot and Cucumber Sticks with Homemade Hummus (V)
Dinner:	Butternut Squash and Chicken Curry (V)

28-DAY MEAL PLAN SHOPPING LIST

Week 1: Day 1 to Day 7

- **Fruits/Veggies:** Bananas, Blueberries, Lemons, Cherry Tomatoes, Pineapple, Pears, Spinach, Tomatoes, Beef
- **Grains:** Quinoa, Buckwheat, Gluten-free Pasta, Gluten-free Muffins Mix
- **Proteins:** Chicken, Salmon, Eggs, Tuna, Steak
- **Dairy & Alternatives:** Cheddar, Feta Cheese, Lactose-free Yogurt, Ice Cream, Buttercream Frosting, Vanilla Cupcakes
- **Condiments/Spices:** Dill, Thai Basil, Maple Syrup, Cinnamon, Garlic Infused Olive Oil, Chimichurri Sauce, Rosemary, Mint, Vanilla Extract
- **Others:** Chia Seeds, Almond Muffins, Low FODMAP Citrus Panna Cotta, Low FODMAP Raspberry Coconut Macaroons, Low FODMAP Blueberry Pie, Low FODMAP-friendly Lemon Cheesecake, Taco Shells, Chocolate

Week 2: Day 8 to Day 14

- **Fruits/Veggies:** Bananas, Blueberries, Pineapple, Coconut, Spinach, Tomatoes, Lettuce, Zucchini, Lemon, Parsley, Red Bell Peppers, Green Beans, Beef
- **Grains:** Buckwheat, Oats, Gluten-free Waffles
- **Proteins:** Pork, Shrimp, Chicken, Eggs, Steak, Turkey
- **Dairy & Alternatives:** Lactose-free Yogurt, Ice Cream, Almond Milk, Cheesecake, FODMAP-friendly Chocolate Mousse, Peanut Butter
- **Condiments/Spices:** Maple Syrup, Salt, Pepper, Cinnamon, Vanilla Extract, Basil, Olive Oil, Chimichurri Sauce, Rosemary, Herbs
- **Others:** Taco Shells, Greek Salad ingredients (olives, feta cheese, cucumber), Almonds, Low FODMAP Citrus Panna Cotta, Low FODMAP Raspberry Coconut Macaroons, Low FODMAP Almond Muffins, Rice, Chia Seeds

Week 3: Day 15 to Day 21

- **Fruits/Veggies:** Strawberries, Apples, Pineapple, Bell Peppers, Broccoli, Tomatoes, Bacon, Eggs, Butternut Squash, Eggplant, Zucchini, Blueberries, Raspberries, Quinoa, Spinach, Rhubarb, Garlic
- **Grains:** Oatmeal, Gluten-Free Bread, Sourdough Bread
- **Proteins:** Tofu, Turkey, Swiss Cheese, Cod, Beef, Shrimp, Halibut, Salmon, Grilled Tuna Steaks
- **Dairy & Alternatives:** Almond Milk, Low FODMAP Mint Chocolate Chip Ice Cream, FODMAP-friendly Lemon Cheesecake, Buttercream Frosting, Simple Vanilla Cupcakes
- **Condiments/Spices:** Cinnamon, Olive Tapenade, Tomato Basil, Sesame Ginger, Dill Sauce, Lemon Herb Sauce, Garlic Infused Olive Oil, Maple Glaze
- **Others:** Chocolate, Low FODMAP Citrus Panna Cotta, Low FODMAP Raspberry Coconut Macaroons, Brown Sugar, Shortbread, FODMAP-friendly Chocolate Mousse, Low FODMAP Maple Oatmeal Cookies, Pineapple Coconut Popsicles, Low FODMAP Blueberry Pie, Chia Seeds

Week 4: Day 22 to Day 28

- **Fruits/Veggies**: Raspberries, Green Beans, Strawberries, Rhubarb, Bananas, Pineapple, Bell Peppers, Lemon, Zucchini, Blueberries, Quinoa, Spinach, Chia Seeds
- **Grains**: Quinoa, Gluten-Free Bread, Rice, Oatmeal
- **Proteins**: Beef, Shrimp, Chicken, Eggs, Tuna
- **Dairy & Alternatives**: Almond Milk, Low FODMAP Raspberry Sorbet, Low FODMAP Citrus Panna Cotta, Low FODMAP Raspberry Coconut Macaroons, FODMAP-friendly Lemon Cheesecake, Buttercream Frosting, Low FODMAP Mint Chocolate Chip Ice Cream
- **Condiments/Spices**: Thai Basil, Garlic, Lemon Garlic, Thyme, Tomato Basil, Lemon Vinaigrette
- **Others**: FODMAP-friendly Chocolate Chip Cookies, Strawberry Rhubarb Crumble, Low FODMAP Blueberry Pie, Chocolate, Brown Sugar, Shortbread, FODMAP-friendly Chocolate Mousse, Low FODMAP Maple Oatmeal Cookies, Simple Vanilla Cupcakes

---

28-DAY VEGETARIAN AND VEGAN MEAL PLAN SHOPPING LIST

Week 1: Day 1 to Day 7

- **Fruits and Vegetables:** Bananas, Strawberries, Blueberries, Zucchinis, Bell Peppers (assorted colors), Carrots, Cucumbers, Avocado, Cherry Tomatoes, Butternut Squash, Broccoli, Raspberries, Lemon, Spaghetti Squash, Assorted Veggies for Grilling (E.g., Bell Peppers, Zucchini, Eggplant, Mushrooms, Onions), Acorn squashes, Kale
- **Grains:** Buckwheat Flour, Quinoa, Gluten-Free Bread, Gluten-Free Pasta, Gluten-Free Waffles
- **Protein:** Tofu, Eggs, Almond Milk
- **Dairy:** Feta Cheese, Lactose-Free Yogurt
- **Nuts and Seeds:** Chia Seeds, Assorted Nuts for Granola (E.g., Almonds, Walnuts)
- **Seasonings and Other:** Sesame, Ginger, Dill, Tomato Basil Sauce, Garlic Infused Olive Oil, Chili, Lemon, Thyme, Chickpeas, Tahini, Olive Oil, Lemon Juice, Garlic, Maple Syrup, Olive Tapenade, Fresh parsley, Nutritional yeast

Week 2: Day 8 to Day 14

- **Fruits and Vegetables:** Bananas, Strawberries, Blueberries, Zucchinis, Bell Peppers (distinct colors), Carrots, Cucumbers, Avocado, Cherry Tomatoes, Butternut Squash, Broccoli, Raspberries, Assorted Veggies for Grilling (E.g., Bell Peppers, Zucchini, Eggplant, Mushrooms, Onions), Lettuce, Acorn squashes, Kale
- **Grains:** Quinoa, Gluten-Free Bread, Gluten-Free Pasta, Gluten-Free Waffles
- **Protein:** Tofu, Eggs
- **Dairy:** Feta Cheese, Lactose-Free Yogurt
- **Nuts and Seeds:** Chia Seeds, Assorted Nuts for Granola (E.g., Almonds, Walnuts)
- **Seasonings and Other:** Sesame, Ginger, Dill, Tomato Basil Sauce, Garlic Infused Olive Oil, Chili, Lemon, Thyme, Chickpeas, Tahini, Olive Oil, Lemon Juice, Garlic, Maple Syrup, Fresh parsley, Nutritional yeast

Week 3: Day 15 to Day 21

- **Fruits and Vegetables:** Bananas, Strawberries, Blueberries, Zucchinis, Bell Peppers (different colors), Carrots, Cucumbers, Avocado, Cherry Tomatoes, Butternut Squash, Broccoli, Raspberries, Lemon, Spaghetti Squash, Assorted Veggies for Grilling (E.g., Bell Peppers, Zucchini, Eggplant, Mushrooms, Onions), Acorn squashes, Kale
- **Grains:** Buckwheat Flour, Quinoa, Gluten-Free Bread, Gluten-Free Pasta, Gluten-Free Waffles
- **Protein:** Tofu, Eggs, Almond Milk
- **Dairy:** Feta Cheese, Lactose-Free Yogurt
- **Nuts and Seeds:** Chia Seeds, Assorted Nuts for Granola (E.g., Almonds, Walnuts)
- **Seasonings and Other:** Sesame, Ginger, Dill, Tomato Basil Sauce, Garlic Infused Olive Oil, Chili, Lemon, Thyme, Chickpeas, Tahini, Olive Oil, Lemon Juice, Garlic, Maple Syrup, Olive Tapenade, Fresh parsley, Nutritional yeast

Week 4: Day 22 to Day 28

- **Fruits and Vegetables:** Bananas, Strawberries, Blueberries, Zucchinis, Bell Peppers (assorted colors), Carrots, Cucumbers, Avocado, Cherry Tomatoes, Butternut Squash, Broccoli, Raspberries, Lemon, Spaghetti Squash, Assorted Veggies for Grilling (E.g., Bell Peppers, Zucchini, Eggplant, Mushrooms, Onions), Acorn squashes, Kale
- **Grains:** Buckwheat Flour, Quinoa, Gluten-Free Bread, Gluten-Free Pasta, Gluten-Free Waffles
- **Protein:** Tofu, Eggs, Almond Milk
- **Dairy:** Feta Cheese, Lactose-Free Yogurt
- **Nuts and Seeds:** Chia Seeds, Assorted Nuts for Granola (E.g., Almonds, Walnuts)
- **Seasonings and Other:** Sesame, Ginger, Dill, Tomato Basil Sauce, Garlic Infused Olive Oil, Chili, Lemon, Thyme, Chickpeas, Tahini, Olive Oil, Lemon Juice, Garlic, Maple Syrup, Olive Tapenade, Fresh parsley, Nutritional yeast

WEIGHT

IMPERIAL	METRIC
1/2 oz	15 g
1 oz	29 g
2 oz	57 g
3 oz	85 g
4 oz	113 g
5 oz	141 g
6 oz	170 g
8 oz	227 g
10 oz	283 g
12 oz	340 g
13 oz	369 g
14 oz	397 g
15 oz	425 g
1 lb	453 g

MEASUREMENT

CUP	ONCES	MILLILITERS	TABLESPOONS
8 cup	64 oz	1895 ml	128
6 cup	48 oz	1420 ml	96
5 cup	40 oz	1180 ml	80
4 cup	32 oz	960 ml	64
2 cup	16 oz	480 ml	32
1 cup	8 oz	240 ml	16
3/4 cup	6 oz	177 ml	12
2/3 cup	5 oz	158 ml	11
1/2 cup	4 oz	118 ml	8
3/8 cup	3 oz	90 ml	6
1/3 cup	2.5 oz	79 ml	5.5
1/4 cup	2 oz	59 ml	4
1/8 cup	1 oz	30 ml	3
1/16 cup	1/2 oz	15 ml	1

TEMPERATURE

FARENHEIT	CELSIUS
100 °F	37 °C
150 °F	65 °C
200 °F	93 °C
250 °F	121 °C
300 °F	150 °C
325 °F	160 °C
350 °F	180 °C
375 °F	190 °C
400 °F	200 °C
425 °F	220 °C
450 °F	230 °C
500 °F	260 °C
525 °F	274 °C
550 °F	288 °C

1. What is a low FODMAP diet?

The Low-FODMAP diet is a dietary approach developed by researchers at Monash University to manage symptoms of Irritable Bowel Syndrome (IBS). It focuses on reducing the intake of certain carbohydrates known to cause digestive discomfort.

2. How does the low-FODMAP Diet work?

The diet restricts high-FODMAP foods that may be poorly absorbed in the small intestine and trigger symptoms in those with IBS. After an elimination phase, reintroduce these foods gradually to identify triggers.

3. What are FODMAPs?

FODMAPs are Fermentable Oligosaccharides, Disaccharides, Monosaccharides, and Polyols. They are specific types of carbohydrates found in various foods that can cause digestive discomfort, especially in those with IBS.

4. Can the low-FODMAP Diet help with other gastrointestinal disorders?

While primarily used for IBS, the low-FODMAP diet may also provide symptom relief for other gastrointestinal disorders, such as Crohn's Disease and Ulcerative Colitis. Always consult with a healthcare provider before starting a new diet.

5. Can a low FODMAP diet help with weight loss?

The diet is not for weight loss; it alleviates digestive symptoms. If you have weight loss goals, consult a dietitian for a personalized plan.

6. Is a low FODMAP diet gluten-free?

Not necessarily, but it does restrict foods with wheat, barley, and rye, which contain gluten and are high in FODMAPs.

7. Can vegetarians/vegans follow a low-FODMAP diet?

Yes, vegetarians and vegans can follow a Low-FODMAP diet. The diet can be adapted to suit various dietary preferences while still avoiding high-FODMAP foods. A dietitian can provide specific guidance.

8. How long does it take for a low FODMAP diet to work?

Symptoms may improve within a few days, but it is recommended to follow the diet for 4-6 weeks under a dietitian's guidance. A dietitian can help you understand the diet, plan your meals, and ensure you're getting all the necessary nutrients.

9. Can I eat dairy on a Low FODMAP diet?

Some dairy products are high in lactose, a FODMAP. However, lactose-free dairy products and certain hard cheeses are usually well-tolerated.

10. How can I maintain a social life while following a Low-FODMAP diet?

Planning is key. Research restaurant menus before dining out, communicate your dietary needs to the hosts of social events and consider bringing your own Low-FODMAP snacks to gatherings.

11. Are there any concerns about the low-FODMAP diet?

While the Low-FODMAP diet can be beneficial, it is restrictive and should be followed under the guidance of a healthcare professional or dietitian to ensure nutritional adequacy.

SCAN THE QR CODE
AND
GET YOUR BONUSES
<u>NOW!</u>

Or copy and paste the following link:

https://pietrofiore.aweb.page/p/35e8cab6-2f7f-406a-a702-2143547bc02a

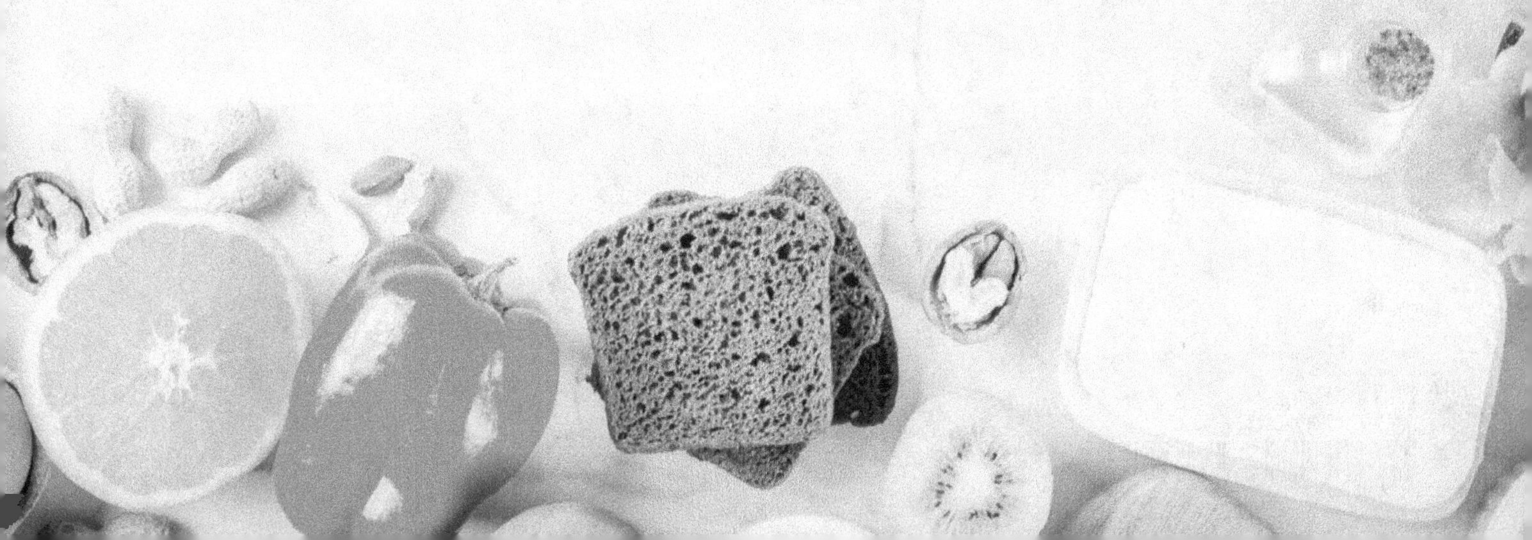

www.ingramcontent.com/pod-product-compliance
Lightning Source LLC
Chambersburg PA
CBHW081554250726
48653CB00009B/3424